How to Stop Smoking in Fifteen Easy Years

A Slacker's Guide to Final Freedom

Other Books By Bear Jack Gebhardt

(See them all on Amazon.com)

Happy John: An Advaita (Non-Duality) Gospel

Practicing the Presence of Peace

The Enlightened Smoker's Guide to Quitting

How to Help Your Smoker Quit

Now Hiring (with Steve Lauer)

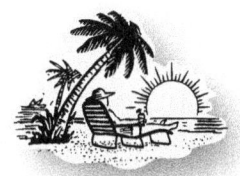

How to Stop Smoking in Fifteen Easy Years

A Slacker's Guide to Final Freedom

Bear Jack Gebhardt

Seven Traditions Press

Fort Collins, Colorado, USA

Copyright © Bear Jack Gebhardt

All Rights Reserved. Published 2012

First Edition

ISBN: **13: 978-1938651021**

Library of Congress: Number: 2012914765

Printed in the United States of America

Material and quotations from *Improv Wisdom: Don't Prepare, Just Show Up*, by Patricia Ryan Madson, Bell Tower Books, 2005, are used with permission from the author, and from the publisher.

For all those who struggle….

Contents

Chapter 1:	Just Be Who You Are …….	1
Chapter 2:	Hop on This Bus	9
Chapter 3:	Easy? How Easy?	15
Chapter 4:	Just Look	22
Chapter 5:	Doing and Not Doing	31
Chapter 6:	The Easiest Way:	41
Chapter 7:	Radical Acceptance	51
Chapter 8:	Easy Homework Check	61
Chapter 9:	More *Ahh* Moments!	68
Chapter 10:	The Hardest Way to Quit:	76
Chapter 11:	A New Lifestyle…	88
Chapter 12:	The Hitchhiker	98
Chapter 13:	Close Up of the Hitchhiker	106
Chapter 14:	Mechanics of Attention	114
Chapter 15:	Mr. T.'s Secret Face	122
Chapter 16:	Step One	130

Chapter 17: Step Two 140

Chapter 18: It's No-Big-Deal 149

Chapter 19: What to Do With Smokes 156

Chapter 20: Hook Me Up Doc 165

Chapter 21: Zyban 175

Chapter 22: Chantix : 182

Chapter 23: Just Make It Up 189

Chapter 24: A Quit Date? 199

Chapter 25: Nourish the Inner Slacker 208

Conclusion... .... 215.

Back of the Bus Dialogues Start on Page ... 217

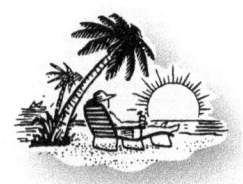

Chapter 1:
Homework Assignment # 1
Just Be Who You Already Are
and Enjoy Your Smokes

"Happiness it the highest spiritual practice."
-- - Rupert Spira

Who you already are is already enough.

We're diving right in on the first page of Chapter One with your first easy homework. I guarantee if you do this first homework it will *immediately* help you start to get unstuck from this silly smoking habit.
 So here's your first homework: ***Just be who you are and enjoy your smokes!*** Got it? I'll repeat: Just be who you *already are* and enjoy your smokes. Yep. That's it. Go ahead, you can start doing your homework right now, if you want. (This book is easy so far, yes?)
 This is the same homework I give when clients call to set a first appointment. I tell them

to stop trying to change things, simply be who they already are and enjoy their smokes. Most of the time they laugh and say okay, that's easy. Sometimes, though, they insist that they don't like being who they are as a smoker and can't enjoy their smokes. So I encourage these folks to at least stop beating themselves up about smoking. (Most smokers beat themselves up all the time about their smoking. And if they don't, someone near them will do it for them.)

If you're going to try me out as your new stop smoking coach and this book as your new how-to-do-it manual, this is your first assignment: Simply be who you are and enjoy your smokes. Questions?

Why Being Yourself and Enjoying Your Smokes is Necessary:

As you'll discover, contrary to what you might assume from that first homework, I really am a professional stop smoking coach, (or smoking cessation counselor, or tobacco treatment specialist, as some stuffed shirts like to call it.) And I was also a long-term smoker who finally quit. So this first homework assignment is not something I just throw at you to make you laugh or get on your good side.

I assume I don't have to explain the first part of the homework--- where you just relax and be yourself. You don't have to be anybody else to quit. Just be yourself--- your ordinary, everyday, non-heroic self. That's the only self that has enough power and wisdom to stop doing the smokes. Besides, as Oscar Wilde put it, "Be yourself. Everybody else is taken."

What may not be quite so apparent is why you should be yourself and also enjoy your smokes. So here are five quick good reasons to enjoy your smokes:

First, because *not* enjoying your smokes and beating yourself up about smoking *doesn't work*! I know this because I've coached clients who have been beating themselves up about their smoking for forty, fifty, even sixty years, and still they smoke. I had one old friend who started smoking at age eight, so he'd been beating himself up, stressing out about smoking for seventy years! But still he smoked. Beating himself up about smoking for most of his long life didn't work. He still hadn't quit!

You, too, may have noticed, if you're currently in need of this book, that stressing out about your smokes hasn't worked yet to help you quit for good. And it probably never will. So let's try something different than stressing out and beating ourselves up about smoking. A different approach might lead to a different result, yes?

The second reason to enjoy your smokes is that it's probably a toss-up as to which habit is worse for your health: smoking, or beating yourself up about your smoking. You may be different but most smokers beat themselves up about their smoking all the time, sometimes all day, every day. Yes, everybody has heard that stress (which is what happens when you beat yourself up) is the number one health hazard we encounter. We know that stress wreaks havoc on our bodies and on our minds in a thousand different ways. But smokers assume that stressing about smoking is *good* stress, politically correct and socially acceptable stress. If you're not stressed about your smoking you're not being a good citizen. You're not taking responsibility.

Wrong. Stress is stress. Stressing about smoking is almost as bad for your health as smoking itself is. That's why your new stop smoking coach says its okay to go ahead, give yourself permission to enjoy your smokes again. To not stress so much about smoking. This is your first homework: Start to *break the habit of beating yourself up about your smokes.*

Granted, you have to be brave to stop stressing about smoking. You're expected to beat yourself up. It is politically and socially correct to feel stressed, guilty, weak, shamed and fearful about your smoking. So if you secretly stop stressing, stop beating yourself up about your smoking, allow yourself to actually *enjoy* smoking, you're going against everything you've been taught, going against your own cultural conditioning.

For most smokers, when they stop beating themselves up about their smoking they are doing something completely different than what they've been doing for many years. Again, if we're going to get different results we need to try something different, yes? For most smokers, not beating themselves up, not stressing is something very different! Welcome to the first taste of final freedom!

The third reason to enjoy your smokes is simply because you can't beat yourself up about smoking and enjoy this book at the same time. And I'd like for you to enjoy this book. If you're like most smokers you're tempted to have a smoke while you read (and while you drive and while you work and while you breathe). So go ahead. Since you're probably going to smoke anyway, you might as well give yourself permission to enjoy it. I don't want you beating yourself up, feeling guilty and sneaky while you're reading this book. If you actually *enjoy* the book, the book is more likely to help you quit smoking, yes? Make sense?

The fourth reason to enjoy your smokes is because we're going to use the same gate to get back out of smoking as we used to get in. Most smokers, when they first started smoking, were just kids, *enjoying* themselves, having an adventure. We were just goofing, having fun, wanting to be in with the in-crowd. When we first started smoking we were following our own natural joy, our secret curiosity and sense of adventure. This is what took us into this habit. Doesn't it make sense to use the same gate --- the same attitudes --- to get back out? Let's *enjoy* ourselves, have fun, be curious while we read this book, maybe even have an adventure while we figure out how to get out of this crazy maze.

And here's **the fifth** and final reason why "enjoying your smokes" is your first homework: because enjoying your smokes is the first step in enjoying *not* smoking. And that's where we're headed: to help you actually *enjoy* not smoking. As you'll discover, it is in the end quite natural, and easy and honest to enjoy not smoking.

In this book you'll discover that quitting smoking, or what I like to call *not doing* your smokes, happens on a particular day, at a particular time and place. However, *enjoying not smoking* is something that stays with you and continues to grow day after day, year after year, no matter where you are. Your joy stays with you. But you have to (get to) *practice* enjoying yourself, just as you are, here from the start, whether you are smoking or not.

I promise that as you read this book you'll learn how to easily, effortlessly, spontaneously enjoy not smoking. You can believe me or not about this promise. Be cynical, if you enjoy to be cynical. But do your homework, then watch, and see what happens.

In this book we will discuss how true freedom really isn't about something as mundane as smoking or not smoking. True freedom is about the capacity, the wisdom to simply enjoy our lives, our *being*, regardless of circumstance, regardless of whether we're smoking or not smoking. **When we're enjoying our lives, we're free. When we're not enjoying, we're chained.**

But I get ahead of myself. For now, just get started on this first easy homework assignment: Relax, be yourself and enjoy your smokes.

Good news: the homework doesn't ever get any harder than this. Welcome to the Slacker's Path!

So go ahead, have a smoke if you want, be yourself and enjoy. You can stop beating yourself up about it. That's step one, and the end of chapter one. Easy so far, yes? We're ready now for chapter two….

Note: At the end of this book you will find "Back of the Bus Questions and Answers" for each chapter, based on real questions real people have asked over the years about the content of each chapter. Most of the "Back of the Bus" sections will be compilations and syntheses from many questioners, though a few will be direct transcriptions of a single questioner's interaction. The "Back of the Bus" Question for this chapter is, *"**How Do I Enjoy My Smokes**?"* which can be found on page 218. You aren't obliged to read it yet, unless of course you enjoy to! I'd suggest instead to just go on to Chapter Two.

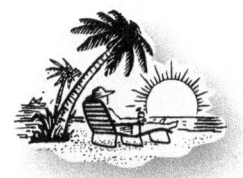

Chapter 2
Where We're Heading:
On the Bus and Off

You're either on the bus or off the bus. If you're on the bus, and you get left behind, then you'll find it again. If you're off the bus in the first place — then it won't make a damn."

—Ken Kesey, as quoted by Tom Wolfe in *The Electric Kool-Aid Acid Test*

I have two passions when it comes to my day job. (My day job now is Head Coach and Chief Janitor at the Smoker's Freedom School. Prior to this, I was a full time stop smoking coach for my county's Health District). My first passion is to figure out how to make quitting smoking easy --- or at least *easier* than most folks tend to make it. And the second is to make this quitting thing, or more precisely, this *freedom* thing, *permanent*. Once we're done, we're *done*. Once we're free, we're free. There's no going back.

Relative to making quitting easy, let me suggest an easy way to read this book is to pretend that you're a tourist in Smoke City (even if you've lived in this city for most of your life) and that you've decided to take one of the tour buses that drive around and show the sites to all the out-of-towners. I'm the guy on the top of the bus, (or inside, if it's raining) with the microphone, pointing out the landmarks. If you're a smoker, you've already paid your dues, you've already bought your ticket. So all you have to do here is sit back, relax, and enjoy the ride. This is a smoker-friendly bus, so you can even enjoy a smoke or two while you ride, if you want. (Again, pretty easy so far, yes?)

So let me take a moment to announce where this bus is going. As our tour bus moves through the Smoke City neighborhoods I'll be pointing out half a dozen or more of the absolutely easiest routes that you might take to get out of this city, e.g., to quit smoking. I've been helping and watching friends and clients slip out of the city, get free, for more than 20 years. They don't all approach the exit using the same streets, same back alleys, or underground tunnels, but a very large percentage of my friends and clients have indeed escaped. So I'll point out many of the routes they've taken. I'll be pointing out signposts, landmarks, estimated travel times and other features of the landscape.

Curiously, however, when it comes to finally getting out of the city, when it comes to

Chapter 2: Where We're Heading

finally quitting smoking, getting free, there's a single off ramp --- let's call it the Easy Exit Off Ramp --- that *every* smoker takes.

Yes, they use a thousand different avenues —a million different avenues --- to finally arrive at this Easy Exit Off Ramp, but it's *this* exit that every single smoker finally must use---and has used--- to successfully get out of the city, and stay out. This whole book offers detailed maps of how to get to the Easy Exit Off Ramp.

According to the Center for Disease Control a million smokers a year successfully quit smoking. Having worked in the trenches, I know smokers approach it —the Easy Exit Off Ramp--- in a million different ways. Maybe they come down Chantix Avenue, or Zyban or Nicotine Patch or Gum Avenue, or Cold Turkey Avenue. Maybe they use Hypnosis Boulevard or come down the "I'm Just Tired of It" Street or "The Doctor Told Me I'd Die If I Didn't Quit" Emergency Lane. One approach often used is, "I Have a New Lover Avenue." It makes no difference which streets they've come down to actually get out of Smoke City. On the final day in which they actually escape Smoke City, *every* smoker slips out via the Easy Exit Off Ramp.

More good news here: the million smokers a year who quit smoking are not all brilliant rocket scientists. Quitting smoking --- walking down the Off Ramp --- is something ordinary people are doing every day.

So on this tour bus we're going to *start* by first quickly making our way to the Easy Exit Off Ramp. We'll drive up and down the surrounding streets where I'll use my author's microphone to point out the coffee shops and rest stops, where it's sunny, where it's shady. I'll point out where many of the other avenues come into and join up with the Off Ramp. We'll even stop the bus and let you walk up and down the streets a bit so you can familiarize yourself with the sights and feelings. We'll drive around the block so you'll know the neighborhood. We're going to make it easy for you to find the Easy Exit Off Ramp.

And then as the tour progresses --- as the book unfolds --- we'll explore some of the outlying areas of the city, driving through some of your old neighborhoods that you're probably familiar with, and have maybe even been lost in, as you've tried to find your way to the Off Ramp.

Although we'll explore the outlying neighborhoods--- looking at various ways people have used and are using to quit smoking, and how they succeed or get stuck --- we'll continually circle around and show how these neighborhoods all hook up to the Off Ramp.

In other words, this book is designed to function as a series of maps to help you get out of Smoke City. These are fun maps. Easy to read maps. But let me say up front here that you don't really need them. You already have within you everything you need to get out of Smoke City. **You don't need a map to get to where you are**! And where you are, as you'll discover, is good enough. You're closer to the Easy Exit Off Ramp than you ever imagined. (That's why "just be who you are" was part of that first homework!)

But I get ahead of myself. I'll try to make this tour bus ride a fun adventure, and very practical and clear and simple enough that you can walk down the ramp and out of Smoke City and never look back. But let me suggest that even if you find my silly metaphors and no-brainer suggestions and somewhat hokey discussions of smoking not to your liking, you can *still* use this book to quit smoking. Smokers have used bright, intelligent and insightful ways to quit smoking, but also have also used the most lame, idiotic, nonsensical avenues to quit smoking.

So you *can* use this book to quit smoking --- whether you consider it bright and insightful or consider it lame and simplistic or somewhere in between. Even if you don't agree with everything (or anything) you find here, you can *still* use it for your own personal reasons. After all, it's not really about this bus --- whether you're off or on. It's about you, and your life, and your freedom. **You don't have to know how to quit smoking before you quit**.

And a final head's up before we get rolling. You will probably find the first part of this ride --- the first part of this book— a bit bumpy and somewhat of an uphill climb as we explore the territory around the Easy Exit Off Ramp. It is so different from other stop smoking books that you may wonder what in the world you signed up for and where it's all going. Trust me on this, as we get into more familiar territory, into your old stomping grounds toward the middle and end of the book, it'll all come together. Your freedom will be so obvious and close you'll settle into it as easily as an old pair of shoes.

Hope you enjoy the ride. Hop aboard…This bus is packed and fueled, engine's started….

[Note: The Back of the Bus discussion for this chapter will be found on page **223**.]

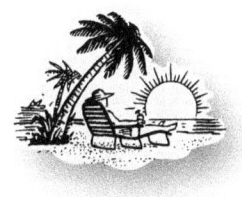

Chapter 3:
Easy? How Easy?
And Why *Fifteen* Years?

"What you learn after you know it all is what counts." -- John Wooden, Hall of Fame basketball player and Hall of Fame coach.

This quit smoking biz is a humbling biz, from both sides of the coin. You have probably already experienced this.

I've noticed that most long term smokers grin and easily resonate with the title, *"How to Stop Smoking in Fifteen Easy Years."* No explanations needed. The title neatly summarizes our history --- and struggles--with smokes.

Younger smokers might relate to the title as a prophetic warning: "Fifteen years happens quicker than you think, kid. No time like the present to get a handle on this thing."

From the other side of the desk, it's been fifteen years since my last stop smoking book was published. Actually, my last two stop smoking books: *The Enlightened Smokers Guide to Quitting* and *How to Help Your Smoker Quit --- A Radically Happy Strategy*. I've been in this biz a while.

Because of those two books--- and because I had been a long time smoker myself, and had been trained and practiced in addiction treatment -- I was hired by our local Health District as a smoking cessation counselor, e.g. a stop smoking coach, or trainer. I've been helping smokers quit for over twenty years.

What I knew about quitting smoking fifteen years ago and what I know now... well, again, to paraphrase Wooden, "It's what you learn after you write the book(s) that can really make a difference."

My first two books were based on what I had learned from my own fifteen year (or more) struggles with quitting, and on what my teachers and trainers had shown me. I assumed I had a handle on the problem. And I did, sort of. *Enlightened Smoker* was distributed in the U.S., Canada, Great Britain, Australia, New Zealand and South Africa, so I had a lot of nice reports from smokers around the world assuring me that the book had helped them walk away from the tobacco wars --- get out of Smoke City. Good. That was my intent.

And then I started sharing and testing those ideas, working one to one with smokers,

Chapter 3::Easy? How Easy?!

and in small groups, day after day, week after week, year after year. What I knew fifteen years ago about smoking was accurate, yes, but only in the same way that what Columbus knew about the new world was accurate. As Shakespeare put it, "There are more things in heaven and earth, Horatio, than are dreamt of in your philosophy."

What I knew fifteen years ago was helpful. Yet only partially so. Let me suggest it may be the same with you. What you already know about smoking and trying to quit is probably mostly true, but if you're still smoking … well, you might find it useful to take a peek at some of these new and more detailed "Exit Maps" that I've put together. I've been a guide on this bus tour for a long time now, thankfully without the weight (and fog) of my own smoking habit. So I've been able to run around a bit, scout out the neighborhood, discover some of the back alleys, recognize the dead ends, the seedy neighborhoods, dangerous parks and easy walking trails. It's the easy walking trails that most interest me. (Like starting with enjoying your smokes!)

You're Not Alone: The Low Success Rates

Alas, a little secret in the stop smoking biz that nobody likes to admit is just how low the success rates are across the country. I don't want to discourage you, but according to the Center for Disease Control the success rate for smokers trying to quit is very low no matter what approach (streets!) they take. The rate stays low whether they're trying it on their own, in a group, over the internet or on the phone, with patches and gum or with Zyban or Chantix or cold turkey. All of these can help — and have helped -- but still the overall success rate for smokers trying to quit is very low --- from 4% to 30%, depending on their methods. Even at 30%, that means seven out of ten smokers wanting to quit don't do it. Uggh.

(If you are independently wealthy, or highly paid and well-insured and have the leisure to take a week or so off to attend the "in-residence" stop smoking program at the Mayo clinic, you might want to do it. At the Mayo in-residence stop smoking clinic your chances of success in quitting go up to almost 50-50. And those, sorry to say, are about the best odds you'll find anywhere in the world for traditional stop smoking programs. Again, and alas, this stop smoking biz, from both sides of the coin, is very humbling.)

From your own experience you probably already know how difficult it is to quit. (You may *already* be discouraged!) The University of Ottawa found that **most smokers try to quit four to seven times over many years before they finally succeed**. That's the bad news.

The good news is that this low success rate in the traditional approaches to stopping smoking ---low even with the help of highly trained and dedicated professionals like those at the Mayo Clinic --- gives us not only the freedom but in fact a <u>mandate</u> to explore radically new approaches--- new paths or trails, new streets, until we find something that actually works to lead us out of Smoke City. We want something that works not just for one or two smokers out of every ten but for nine out of ten. (That tenth guy might need to work on his meth habit before these trails will work for him.) This is, after all, a life and death quest.

Here's more good news: After fifteen years of daily working as a professional stop smoking coach, testing both old and new strategies with friends and clients, I know (in all humility) that I really have found some much easier maps that lead out of these smoky neighborhoods. Or at least easier than most folks, especially folks in the medical community, tend to make it.

I know I've found easy ways to help smokers quit smoking (like enjoying your smokes!) because the government agency for which I worked employed independent evaluators to quantitatively evaluate our programs. They called up my clients seven months after their second session. These evaluators have the numbers to confirm that the maps I've discovered since writing my first books actually *do* help smokers quit more often and more permanently than almost any other program in the country. Yay.

I wish I could say I invented them --- these easy avenues for quitting smoking, and the Easy Exit Off Ramp in particular--- but I didn't, any more than Columbus invented the new world. We credit him because he had map makers with him who allowed others to follow the same journey. Same here. I didn't invent the territory. I'm confident, though, that I have new, more accurate maps than what we've been using.

Nevertheless, what I share in this book are basically reminders of what you already know. And thus, alas, the maps may seem overly obvious. Columbus had the same problem. It seemed overly obvious. "If you're going to explore the new world," Columbus suggested, "you need to sail west." Duh.

Over these past years I've had the pleasure of observing how real smokers actually quit --- most of them long term, pack-a-day or more smokers. We became friends. We talked in depth as they were getting ready to quit, and then again as they actually quit and then again in the days, weeks and months after they quit--- or didn't quit, or quit and went back to smoking before they quit again. I still feel quite honored to be part of this very brave, private and life-changing process.

It doesn't need to take fifteen years. Or another fifteen years. It can happen easily, naturally, joyfully, simply while reading this book. You can *let it* happen this way. Since most people assume that quitting smoking is very hard, very hit and miss, painful and nerve wracking, if you decide you're going to let it be

Chapter 3::Easy? How Easy?!

easy, you have to be brave. **You have to be brave to let it be easy.**

So be brave. Let it be easy. Let's get this bus rolling…

[Note: The Back of the Bus discussion for this chapter will be found on page **224.**]

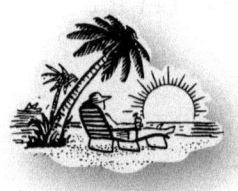

Chapter 4:
Homework Assignment # 2:
Just Look, Observe

"Joy in looking and comprehending is nature's most beautiful gift." --- Albert Einstein

Okay, your first homework assignment was to just be yourself and enjoy your smokes. Your second assignment is to *just look, observe*. (So far, this approach to quitting smoking is a slacker's dream, e.g. really easy, yes?)

So, what to observe?

As I've already mentioned, as we drive around on this bus I will point here and there, suggesting particular places for you to look. Again, I'm the guy with the microphone at the top of the tourist bus pointing out various historical parks, buildings and fire hydrants as we cruise through Smoke City.

But obviously, you're not a tourist in the city of smokes. You actually live here. So when I point out the sights, please, test them against your own experience. This is how we can best work together --- observing our real life, kicking the tires and looking under the hood of our experiences with smoking and not smoking. Test everything you read in this book against your own direct experience.

One of the basic lessons I've learned in over fifteen years in this business is that **you, the smoker are the true expert in what will work best for you to quit**. So again, test everything I say against your own experience. Go slow. Tell the bus driver to stop, if you need to. Stop reading. Get off the bus and look closer at what you see. Once you're satisfied you've seen what there is to see, hop back on. We have time. Fifteen years, if need be.

What We're Looking for: The *Ahh* Moment

So what to observe first? How about a particular, single moment of our smoking experience?

Although we've been talking about quitting in fifteen easy years (which is, according to the Center for Disease Control, how long most smokers take before they actually quit), these years come at us a moment at a time. It's like the old question: how do you eat an elephant? Right. A bite at a time.

So let's start this easy process by looking very closely at a single moment, single bite, of our shared smoking experience. A moment with which almost every smoker can identify.

Here's the set up: Let's say you've been wanting to quit. (Why else would you be reading this book?) If you will, remember one of the last times you tried to quit, especially when you had been doing pretty well, maybe cutting way back or maybe you hadn't smoked at all, for an hour or a day or a week or more. Congrats.

But then, doggone it, something happened. You found yourself in a place where you couldn't get your attention off smokes. The craving for a smoke was so strong that you couldn't think of anything else. You were really *jones'n* for a smoke, *really. really* craving. In fact, you were so tempted that, once again, you gave in, gave up the struggle, found yourself another smoke. In that moment it was obvious, at least to you, that you really, *really* needed a smoke. If you were like most smokers you probably told yourself that it would be just one more, quick, sneaky little smoke, maybe even just a puff or two, to get over that stupid, unrelenting craving. So you caved.

You went out and bought a pack. Or took your old smokes off your night stand, or out of the trash can. Or you asked your spouse, or neighbor or some stranger on the street. One way or another, you found yourself with a smoke in hand. (*"Thank God!"*) You bummed a match, or found your lighter, actually lit the stupid thing, took a deep first inhale, then exhale. *Ahhh*...**back home again**. What a relief!

(Isn't this a neighborhood of Smoke City—a moment in Smoke City--- with which we are all familiar?)

Okay, let's freeze-frame this "*ahh* moment," this back-home-with-a-smoke moment. This is the moment we want to look at more closely because this feeling of relief after that first exhale when we've been denying ourselves is *exactly* what we've been wanting to experience. So let's just look at this moment more closely.

And yes, these "*ahh* moments," these "back-home" moments, don't just come when we've been trying to quit and then we cave in. They also come when we've been in some "forced abstinence" environment, on a long airline flight or at the in-laws or spending a weekend in jail. When we haven't been able to smoke, or haven't allowed ourselves for a while, and finally we get to have a smoke. We finally are in a place where we can light up, so we do and we take that first long drag and first exhale… *ahh… back home…*

Again, a familiar neighborhood in smoke city, yes?

In that *ahh moment* after the first exhale, we're perfect. What a relief. We're right where we want to be. We're complete. Fulfilled. We don't want to be anywhere else. Why?

Let's be clear: Contrary to the easy explanation, **it's *not* in fact the nicotine** (even though we call it a nicotine fit), because the amount of nicotine we get from one little puff is actually quite minimal. I have worked with many smokers who report that even while using the nicotine patch, or nicotine gum or lozenge, they still feel that craving for a smoke (Though maybe not as intensely.) Yet they, too, when they cave and have a smoke, experience that same "*ahh ...*" relief from that first inhale and exhale. For the folks wearing nicotine patches or chewing nicotine gum their nicotine levels are *already* quite sufficient! And even if the nicotine level is low, **one lousy puff is not going to make it go back up again**. But still there's that real, obvious, even sensual "*ahh....*"

So let's look closely and be very clear about this: it's *not* the nicotine that provides the "first puff relief." It must be something else that makes us go, "*ahhh.*" So what is it?

To see it clearly, and put this moment in context let's move now to the second or third puff. With that second or third puff, if we've been wanting to quit, we start to beat ourselves up again. "Oh shoot, here I go again. I'm smoking again! Doggone it. What am I doing? Why am I doing this? I wanted to quit so bad, but here I am smoking again ...*thump, thump thump.*"

Chapter 4: Just Look!

If we haven't necessarily been wanting to quit but are simply resuming the habit after a forced abstinence, **by the second or third puff we're back in the groove again--- same ol' same ol'.** We're probably not even thinking of our smokes anymore, or the forced abstinence. We're thinking about the football game or whether to buy gas or what cousin Lois said about Harry. There's no special *"ahh"* feeling attached to our smokes after the first several puffs. (There are exceptions to the rule, of course, but in general... isn't this your experience?)

So back to the "freeze frame" of the first puff, or more precisely, the *exhale* of the first puff, the *"ahh* moment." Let's look at it more closely. When we look closely, we see that in that moment after that first exhale, we are no longer *wanting* a cigarette because, (duh) we're now smoking one! In fact, we don't want *anything*. In that brief half moment, we are happy to ***just be*** right where we are, doing what we're doing. We are simply *being* what feels like our ordinary selves.

Here's a point on the map that's very important to observe: Most smokers mistakenly assume that the relief they feel came from the cigarette. In fact, however, **the *"ahh"* relief is a relief from** *wanting*. And more precisely, it's the relief of allowing ourselves to simply enjoy the moment, not looking forward or back, *just being our natural selves.* In that *"ahh moment"* we're not *wanting* anything. We're not *doing* anything (except smoking.) We're *just being* present, being ourselves, enjoying the moment, enjoying our smoke.

Alas, starting with the second puff, or the third or fourth, the "wanting" and *doing* start back up again--- this time, *wanting to quit*! Or wanting to go get some gas. Wanting to tell cousin Lois a thing or two. So the relief from the smoke is no longer so sweet. So what often happens, we have another one, and then another one, subconsciously trying to get that "first puff relief," that first "*ahh*." Again though, the **relief did not come from the cigarette**. The relief came because of the *momentary absence of wanting*! The relief came from taking our incessant wanting, or "doing" out of gear and just for one brief moment allowing ourselves to enjoy simply *being here*, even with a smoke, at ease and at rest --- *ahh*.

So, from here at the top of the tour bus, we can see, even if it's just a glimpse in passing, that what we truly "crave," when we cave: the *absence of wanting*! We want to be "want-less!" We want to be *at ease* in the moment. *Ahhh...*

Here's more good news (I promise, this book is full of good news!): You don't have to *do* anything about this insight, or this sight from the top of the bus. You don't have to *do* anything about the "*ahh* moment" except recognize its occasional presence in your life, here in Smoke City.

Again, your homework is to simply look, observe.

Okay, let's look a little deeper. Isn't the *ahh* moment --the *absence of wanting* -- what we also *want* in all the other areas of our lives? Aren't we looking for the *ahh* moment--- the want-less moment --- when we envision being rich, or being in love, or being famous or in perfect health? Aren't we envisioning a state where all of our *wants* have all been met? We can envision lying on a tropical beach in our perfect body next to our perfect lover, supported by our perfect bank account which came from our perfect job. And of course, our perfect family and perfect friends are all watching on admiringly. In such a scenario all of our *wants* are met! *Ahh*, success.

Again, what we've been doing here is simply isolating a single moment of our smoking lives--- the *"ahh moments"*--- and observing that the relief we experience in these moments is **a relief from wanting**. A willingness to *just be* who we already are in the moment.

With this observation under our belt, we're ready to lay the ground work, set the stage for the "Number One Absolutely Easiest Way to Quit Smoking. "

Before we get to the absolutely easiest way to quit, though, we'll need to look again at the map and the territory around the Easy Exit

Ramp. For that we'll need another chapter. And maybe another smoke, if you be so moved ... *Ahh...*

[Note: The Back of the Bus discussion for this chapter will be found on page **225.**]

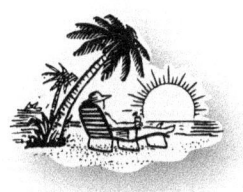

Chapter Five:
The Neighborhood Leading to
The Easy Exit Off-Ramp

"There seems to be some perverse human characteristic that likes to make easy things difficult." --- Warren Buffet

We'll start here and in the next couple of chapters mapping out the absolutely easiest way to get to the Easy Exit Off Ramp, e.g., the easiest way to quit smoking. I give more time and attention to these first maps, these first approaches simply because --- well, they're easiest, and they actually work to help folks quit smoking.

Nevertheless, at first glance these first maps might seem a bit strange, or complicated, hard to follow. That's only because these aren't the usual maps you commonly find in other stop smoking programs. In other words, we'll discuss things, observe things here in this and the next couple of chapters that aren't generally observed or discussed in other approaches to quitting smoking. (Like the "*ahh* moment.") Even though this approach is unusual let's remember that according to the Center for Disease Control, the other approaches, the other off-ramps, generally *fail* for seven or eight or even nine out of every ten smokers who try them. So stick with me. We'll go slow so you can familiarize yourself with the territory. Make your way step by step to the very workable Easy Exit Off-Ramp.

As I said, these first maps lay out the easiest way to quit smoking. In fact, they show you how you can discover freedom from smokes in less than a second. To get to that place, however, we must cut through a lot of accumulated underbrush and overgrown clinging vines.

But let me forewarn you: very few of us are brave enough to let quitting smoking (or our lives!) be transformed so quickly and easily. **Most of us just aren't trained (yet) to let freedom come that easily.** So don't worry if you don't quit smoking in the next couple of chapters. Stick with the program. It *will* happen by the end of the book.

Since most of us *aren't* ready to let it be so easy, after these first chapters we'll drive the bus back into more familiar territory, cruising (rather quickly) past the hospital, then the nursing home and then the hospice center to look briefly at the maps for the absolutely *hardest* ways to quit smoking. **(In a nutshell, the** absolutely hardest way to quit, contrary to popular opinion, is in response to worries about our physical health.)

After a quick drive past the hospital and nursing homes we'll get back to exploring and mapping out the much easier, more fun and natural ways to quit. On their own, any one of these maps can lead you to the Off Ramp. Put together, overlaid, these maps work even better. So just ride along. Don't worry about when or how to quit smoking. It'll happen. Just watch. But enough of the introductions. Let's get to it.

The Easy Exit Off Ramp:

The Single Exit *Every* Smoker Uses to Quit:

As I've already mentioned, and as you'll discover, each of the hundreds of millions of smokers throughout history who have ever quit smoking did it (in essence) in the exact same way --- using the Easy Exit Off Ramp. I know that's a bold statement. Smokers themselves might disagree. But I stand by it. I guarantee that in essence, *all* the ways boil down to this first, most simple of ways. So let's dive in, cut some underbrush.

In the last chapter we looked at the "*ahh* moment" – that moment after the first inhale and exhale when we're at ease. Set the "*ahh* moment" aside for a moment. We'll come back to it shortly.

Let's look now at the act of smoking itself. Smoking, if you will observe, is something that we *do*, both consciously and unconsciously, for a hundred or a thousand different reasons. We "do" smoking not only with our hands, our lips and our lungs, but also with our eyes, ears, thoughts, feelings, sensations. Smoking is something that we are *doing*, whether we are doing it actively, while actually sucking in and blowing out smoke, or passively, when we're briefly thinking about how long it's been since our last smoke, or when we will have the next smoke, or checking to see how many smokes we have left, thinking about where next to smoke, when to smoke, etc.

Again, not meaning to be too simplistic, but in order to point out the absolutely easiest way to quit smoking it's important to first point out --- to observe --- that smoking is something that we *do*, or, more precisely, that *you* do. Again, *duh*.

Okay, now, let's look closely. Although smoking is something that you do, **quitting smoking is *not* fundamentally something that you *do*.** Quitting smoking is something you *cease* **doing,** stop doing. In essence, at it's very heart, quitting smoking is *not* something that anybody anywhere in the world has ever *done*. Quitting smoking is simply *not doing* the smokes! (That's what the hundreds of millions of smokers who have quit smoking all have in common!)

This is not just word games. Although quite simple, this is actually a very powerful observation. (So I'll stop the bus here for a moment, and repeat it, again put it in bold.) **Quitting smoking is not something that you do. It's something that you _cease_ doing.**

And there's the rub: many smokers find that smoking is something they **can't stop _doing!_** When friends or family ask, "Why don't you just quit?" what they mean is "Why don't you _just stop doing_ it? But smokers report they _can't_ stop _doing_ it! How curious.

It gets even more curious. When smokers find they can't stop _doing_ their smokes, they start looking around for something that they can _do_ that might help them stop _doing_ the smoking! So they _do_ hypnosis or _do_ cutting back or _do_ nicotine patches or gum or they _do_ toothpicks, carrots, a cabin in the mountains, herbal concoctions, deep breathing, eye exercises or a mixture of all these, hoping that they can find something to _do_ that will help them stop _doing_ their smokes.

Alas, for many smokers nothing they _do_ seems to work to help them stop _doing_ their smokes, at least for very long. Yes? You can see this? You can see that we are trying to _do_ something to help us stop _doing_ something else?

Okay. Back on the bus.

To repeat (because it's important to understand the easiest way to stop smoking):

We've just looked at how smoking is something that we *do*, and that quitting smoking is not something we *do* but rather something we *cease* doing. And we've looked at how we so often look for something we can personally *do* that will help us stop *doing* smokes! (Don't worry if this sounds confusing. You don't have to *do* anything here except observe what's being pointed out. You don't have to *do* anything about any of these observations. Stick with the homework: just observe, and enjoy).

So okay, now let's take a quick look at *doing*. (This is all leading to the absolutely easiest way to quit smoking, I promise. Just stay on the bus. We're almost there.)

When we were very young kids --- from age two to age four or five --- we were *doing* all day long, running here, there, playing with this, playing with that. But we weren't too personally concerned with the outcome of any of our *doing*. You could set us down in front of a pile of rocks, or some cardboard boxes, and we'd be happy to sit and *do* rocks or cardboard for a while.

Although as young kids we were *doing* all day long, our focus wasn't actually on the *doing*; it was on simply *being kids*. Or more precisely, simply *being*. And for 98% of us, this *just being* (as a kid) was magical. At that age, the world was wide open and wonderful, full of beautiful colors, living mysteries and everyday items of tangible deliciousness. *Just being* here alive on this planet was enough!

Of course, since we were just kids we had very little control over any of this. Big people could literally pick us up and move us from one spot to another. They would tell us what to wear, what to eat, where to go, what to say, what to think, sometimes gently, often times not. Still, as a kid—just *being* a kid, *just being*—was absolutely perfect, (except for what the adults were *doing* to us, or forced us to *do*.) In general, as kids we were simply alive and aware and didn't know we needed anything else for our well-being but to simply *be present*.

And then by about age five or six, when we started first grade, our attention was directed more and more to personal *doing*. "Okay children, today we are going to *do* spelling, and then *do* arithmetic." We started to learn that our well-being depended on how well we personally could *do* spelling, or personally *do* arithmetic.

Throughout our school years, fourth, fifth, sixth, eighth grade, this basic lesson was repeated time and again. **Our well-being depended on what we were personally *doing*, and what we were personally *not doing*.** ("Do your homework, don't do so much daydreaming.")

The same lesson was being handed out at home. We learned that our well-being depended on what we did or didn't do. "Do the dishes, don't do that to the cat, do your room, don't do that to your food."

By the time we were in high school this basic lesson was ingrained and automatic. ("Your well-being depends on what you personally *do* and/or don't do.") The cool people were the ones who were personally *doing* the cool things—playing on the football team or being on the cheerleading squad, or for other segments, personally *doing* the chess club, or the pool hall or the car shows.

For most of us, this is when we started personally *doing* smokes. "Doing smokes" is what cool people did. Or the rebels. Or just our regular friends. We started personally *doing* smokes in order to achieve, or express, our own personal coolness, to express our own personal well-being here in the world.

When when we finally left school -- whether after 8th grade or after earning a Ph.D -- that old basic lesson (what you *do* determines your well-being) became even more intense, more obvious. When we went to work we were paid to *do* certain things. If we did them, our well-being increased. If we didn't do them, our well-being decreased.

Here in our adulthood the ubiquitous religious faith throughout the world is "faith in personal *doing*" to bring about well-being. It's not totally wrong. We have accumulated evidence for the efficacy of such faith. When we *do* our laundry, we have achieved "personal laundry well-being" for the week. But after we *do* the laundry, we think we next need to *do* the dishes, or *do* the vacuuming, *do* the climbing of Mount Everest, *do* the discovery for the cure for cancer, and the lawn needs mowing. We are all, all of the time, *doing, doing, doing* with the hope, the faith that by enough *doing* we will achieve, establish our well-being.

But if you will notice **this *doing, doing, doing* is an unending cycle.** Some of us need a break. So we stop *doing* for a moment and have a smoke. We stop *doing*, light one up. Exhale… *Ahh…* there, just for a moment, well-being.

But no. We're so addicted to *doing, doing*, we have such great faith in our *doing* to bring about well-being, that we automatically start *doing* stuff again, even while we're smoking. Maybe we do a crossword puzzle, or talk on the phone. While we smoke we *do* stuff with our thoughts and our talk, if not with our hands and our walk. So we don't experience the relief we were looking for—the relief from *doing* all the time. So, still looking for relief, we light up another one.

Again, you don't have to *do* anything about this description of the smoking cycle. Just observe, and enjoy. By now you probably see where we're going. You sense what the "absolutely easiest way to quit smoking" might be. You sense, correctly, that the Easy Exit Off

Ramp might be very close at hand. And it is. But for that, let's *do* another chapter...

[Note: The Back of the Bus discussion for this chapter will be found on page **227**]

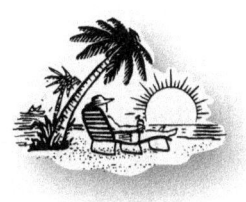

Chapter 6:
The Absolutely Easiest Way to Quit:
Just Be
and *Do* What You're Already *Doing*!

The snow goose need not bathe to make itself white. Neither need you do anything but be yourself

---LaoTzu

On this bus we occasionally have to go around the block to see again what we just saw. So let me repeat: Smoking is something we personally *do*. But (here's more good news) *quitting* smoking is not something we can ever personally *do*. Quitting smoking is actually quite impersonal. Quitting smoking is something we simply *cease doing*, just like we cease our personal bungee jumping, or cease our personal cliff diving, cease running guns to the Uruguayan Tupamaro guerrillas.

Question: What do you have to *do* to no longer bungee jump or no longer dive off a cliff or no longer smuggle guns? Right, you don't *do* anything! Nothing personal about it! To not do these things you can allow yourself to *be a slacker*! Don't do *anything*!

So how do we stop *doing* our personal smokes? Here's the key: We don't need to *do* anything! Again, smoking is something we *do*. Quitting smoking is something we *cease* doing.

So instead of focusing on our *doing*, we shift our focus just an inch and allow ourselves to *not do*, to simply *be*, for the moment, without *doing* smokes. **We allow ourselves to be who we are already being in that moment** --- whether it's jumpy or peaceful. And even more deliciously, we can allow ourselves to actually *enjoy just being*, (be it jumpy or peaceful) for that brief moment. *Ahh…*

Time and again I have worked with smokers who have been trying to *do* something about their smoking for many years but have somehow become stuck. Some have cut down to two or three smokes a day, but can't make the final drop. Others have cut down from smoking a pack or two packs a day to a half a pack or less. They feel that they have run into a wall, so to speak. Just can't seem to actually cut free. What to *do*?

And of course I've worked with many smokers who haven't cut down at all, but they've been *wanting* to quit for years --- maybe decades --- but can't even *start* to quit. They want to know where to start? How to *do* it?

They all feel that at some point, the Nike motto "*Just Do It*!" is appropriate. Most smokers who get stuck, who can't "just do it," are very caught up in *thinking* about their smoking, and not smoking. Or are very caught up in the feelings surrounding their smoking and not smoking. **Smokers get caught up in their thoughts and feelings, worries and fears about smoking and not smoking**. (Sound familiar?) It's useful to recognize that all of these thoughts and feelings, worries and fears are in themselves *doings*!

It's freeing to recognize that at some point more thoughts, more feelings, more strategies, more waiting and wondering are simply *not* useful. Many smokers have been fussing over quitting smoking for fifteen years or more. They get to a point where it really is time to "just do it." You yourself may be at this point right now!

Good news here again. To repeat: smoking is something that we *do*. Quitting smoking is, in essence, *not* something that we *do*. Quitting smoking is something that we *cease* doing. So curiously, when we come to that point where it's time to "*just do it*," just quit smoking, completely, totally, once and for all, **there is nothing we have to do**! No particular action. No particular thought. No particular feeling. We don't need more courage. Or strength. Or insight. We just do it. Or more precisely, we just don't do it. We don't *do* smokes. Just like we don't smuggle guns to Central America or don't bungee jump. When it comes to *doing* smokes, we finally just give ourselves permission to be slackers.

And then we let whatever happens happen because of our slacker approach. We let all the thoughts, feelings, sensations or experiences happen that are going to happen. And more good news: We don't have to *do* anything about these, either. We can allow ourselves to be slackers in regard to *everything* related to smoking!

To quit smoking, we don't have to *do* anything! Again, quitting smoking is not something that we *do*. It's something we *cease* doing. (Have I said it enough times -- pointed it out enough times -- that it's starting to crack the "Just do it" worldview with which we have all been brainwashed?)

Yes, when we *cease doing our smokes* many thoughts, feelings, sensations are going to rise up in us. Believe it or not, many of these thoughts, feelings and sensations that rise up after we simply *cease doing* our smokes will be quite pleasant, quite comfortable. Other thoughts, feelings and sensations that rise up after *not doing* smokes may not be so comfortable. Either way, we don't have to *do* anything about any of these thoughts, feelings or sensations that rise up, be they comfortable or uncomfortable. We can be slackers, because whatever rises up will also fall away, on its own. That's how life works, both inside and out.

And so again, at some point, for every smoker, the planning and plotting and waiting and thinking and worrying and delaying and strategizing about quitting is over. It's time. Right now. *Just do it*! Do what? Be a slacker! *Do nothing*! Just don't do smokes! And let the chips fall where they may.

What all smokers discover when they actually quit *doing* smokes is that *not doing smokes* is actually much easier, much simpler, much more peaceful and natural then they had ever imagined!

But you don't have to think about what it's going to be like after you "don't do it." That's just more fussing, more worrying, more strategizing. The only thing you need to *do* right now --- *just don't do anything!* Just don't pick up the smokes, then let what happens happen. Instead of *doing* anything, *just be* for a moment, and go on about your life.

To not *do* anything, and *just be* who you already are without the smokes is the absolutely easiest way to quit smoking.

Who you already are without the smokes is the real you, the natural you. That's why it's the easiest way to quit. You don't have to *be* anybody different. And you don't have to *do* anything!

One more piece of good news before we close the chapter: **You are already "just being"** who you already are without the smokes. You're *already being* the natural you. You don't have any choice about it!

Again, just look, observe. Your body is already being your body, with or without smokes! And your mind continues to be your mind, with or without smokes. You don't have to *do* anything about your body or your mind! Let them *do* what they naturally *do*, while you just *be* with them.

Yes, of course, different sensations, urges, icky-ness and pleasures come and go in the body, rise and fall, whether you're smoking or not smoking. And your mind judges these sensations as good and bad, tolerable or intolerable, pleasant or unpleasant. Again, you don't have to *do* anything about your body or mind. *Just b*e with them. And more specifically, *just be* who you already are without *doing* smoking.

Just being who you already are without doing smokes is in fact very natural, very easy, even effortless. Again, that's why it's the absolutely easiest way to quit smoking! You don't have to *do* anything!

So how do we stop *doing* our smokes and allow ourselves to simply *be*, for a moment?

Piling on the good news: *Just being* without smokes is not something we *do*! We are already doing it! We are already *just being*. It's our natural state. Our deepest state. Our free state!

So we simply give ourselves permission to *be* without smokes wherever we happen to be. We give ourselves permission to simply *not do* smoking and *be* who we already are in that moment, whoever that happens to be. We give ourselves permission to take our focus off of *doing*, for just a brief moment and simply enjoy being. *Ahh…*

Our ordinary *being* is in fact quite powerful. Our basic, ordinary *being* is the source and substance of our physical and mental energy. When we remember and honor our simple, basic *being*, even for very brief moments, we energize our body and our mind; we energize our whole existence. Our *doing* doesn't stop. But *doings* come and go. *Doings* include all our thoughts, feelings, sensations and worries. Our *ordinary being* is something we can remember, and rely on in every moment. That's why **our *being* is so much more reliable for helping us quit smoking than are our *doings*.**

And when we look at it closely, we can observe that *"not-doing smokes, just being"* is the single simple step that *every* smoker takes to quit smoking, whether he or she recognizes it or not. Many, maybe even most, ex-smokers do not necessarily recognize that this is the simple step that they took to quit smoking. Still, we can observe: **this "not doing" is the essence of quitting smoking**!

But around the world we are all very focused on *doing, doing*. It's the basic religion, where we all place our faith. Everyone is so identified with *doing* that when smokers are asked how they quit smoking they will focus on what they were *doing* when they stopped *doing* smokes.

"I chewed a lot of gum, I painted the house, I ran, I meditated, I prayed, I cried, I slept, I snapped a rubber band, I yelled at my cat." All of these things may indeed have been "done," but at root, in essence, what every single smoker actually "did" was stop *doing* the smokes. They each allowed themselves to be free of that *doing*. They allowed themselves to be a slacker when it came to doing smokes!

By allowing ourselves to *just be* whoever we happen to be in the moment, the chain reactions around *doing* start to subside. When we allow ourselves to *just be*, we begin to spontaneously master our doings, not only with smoking, but also in every other arena of our lives.

Just being who we already are without smokes is in fact quite peaceful. And it's easy. And because we are remembering our *being*, this practice is also very energizing, as well as quite creative, entertaining and empowering. To *stop doing* our smokes we allow our thoughts, feelings and sensations to "do" whatever they do while for brief moments we just "be" with them. We don't try to stop all the *doings*. We simply move our attention — move our loyalty, our emphasis — off of *doing* and onto *being*. In *just being*, we find freedom.

***Just being* who we already are is the easiest way to *stop doing* smoking, if we are brave enough to "do it."**

Obviously, for many people this *stop doing, just be* seems "too simple," too easy, even heretical. After all, most smokers have been searching for years and years for something they can *do* to stop smoking. To suggest *stop doing, just be who you already are* may appear too obvious, almost insulting, or at least embarrassing. It's like telling our friend who is looking for her glasses --- they're on the top your head. Oh yea.

So, although *stop doing, just be* is the absolutely easiest way to quit smoking, in the next chapter we'll make the process a little more complicated. We still want the process to be easy, of course, but if we need a little more meat we can give ourselves something to *do* in order to *stop doing, just be*.

So okay --- let's move to the second easiest way to quit smoking. It's not actually different than this first easiest way, but it (sorta) gives us something to *do* while we are *not doing* our smokes and just being. Onwards. Let's *just be* while we *do* the next chapter!

[Note: The Back of the Bus discussion for this chapter will be found on page **228.**]

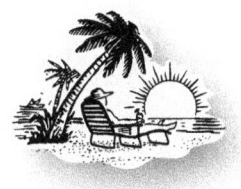

Chapter 7

The Second Easiest Way to Quit: Radical Acceptance

Happiness can exist only in acceptance.
                                                  --- George Orwell

    I suspect I've been overloading some of you lifelong cynics with too much good news, so to balance things out I'm now obliged to give you some bad news. Here it is:

    The various easy ways to quit smoking (in fifteen easy years) that are outlined in this book are not completely different exits. As I've already mentioned, if you are ever going to quit smoking, you will have to sneak out using the Easy Exit Off Ramp

    In other words, if at some point you don't simply *stop doing* your smokes and be brave enough to *just be who you already are,* you will never quit smoking. Never. Ever. Sorry, that's just the way life works.

At some point, even if it's not until you are on your death bed, you will indeed stop doing smokes and *just be* who you already are. When you stop *doing* smokes, you are no longer a smoker. (Duh.)

No smoker, anywhere in the world, at any time in history, has escaped "doing" this first basic technique. Every single smoker who has ever quit at some point simply *stopped doing* his or her smokes and allowed himself or herself to *just be* whoever he or she happened to be in that moment.

Yes, of course, you can choose from a whole circus of tricks about what you might *do* both before and after you *stop doing* smokes. Nevertheless, the single, essential, mandatory piece of the quitting process is that at some point you will simply *stop doing* your smokes, no matter what else you choose to *do*. That's actually good news and a lot simpler than we tend to make it.

And yes, again, when you *stop doing* your smokes a whole rainbow of thoughts, feelings, sensations and actions will rise up in your being, just as a whole rainbow of thoughts, feelings, sensations and actions rises up as you *continue* doing your smokes. Such a rainbow of sensations is with us every single moment! Life goes on, whether you are *doing* smokes or not.

Chapter 7: The 2nd Easiest Way to Quit

You may plan some of your actions, some of your thoughts, feelings and sensations around the time you *stop doing* smokes. For example, you might plan to practice deep breathing and/or chewing nicotine gum, and/or long baths and/or staying away from Aunt Martha who smokes like a chimney. Plans are fine, maybe even necessary. We'll offer some fun plans and useful techniques for this time of "not doing" as this book unfolds.

Nevertheless, regardless of what you *plan* for the time around when you *stop doing* your smokes, most of the thoughts, feelings, sensations and actions that rise up in you will be quite spontaneous and effortless, *unplanned*, just as they are prior to quitting.

As we've already discussed, most of the thousands of stop smoking methods offered to smokers today are all focused on what a smoker should *do* before, during and after he or she *stops doing* the smokes. Again, these *doings* can indeed be helpful. I myself collected over a hundred different *doings* to help my friends and clients *stop doing* smokes before I finally recognized that in essence quitting smoking is *not* something we *do*. Quitting smoking is something we *cease* doing.

So (I can't help myself) here's some more good news: If we focus first on the very *essence*, the fundamental *act* of quitting smoking — which is simply *not doing* the smokes --- it makes the whole process so much more understandable and thus so much easier.

At some point in this journey away from smokes you will find yourself engaging "the absolutely easiest way to quit smoking"--- e.g., you will find yourself *not doing smokes* and *just being* who you already naturally are. As you'll discover when it comes to the actual experience of this *not doing*, it is not really difficult to be such a slacker. In fact, it's quite enjoyable. It's a little bit like someone telling you, "At some point, you're going to have to eat that piece of cheese cake," or "At some point, you're going to have to cash that thousand dollar check."

Ahh, cheese cake. *Ahh*, a thousand bucks. *Not doing* smokes and just being who we already are really can be, really *is*, a wonderful gift we give ourselves.

But I get ahead of myself.

The second easiest way to quit smoking goes hand in glove with the first. It's a simple reminder that helps us *do* the first. It's called Radical Acceptance. Again, as with the first easiest way *(stop doing smokes, just be who you already are)*, it will take me much longer to explain Radical Acceptance and put it into context than it takes for you to *do* it. In fact, you *do it* --- this radical acceptance --- in one brief moment.

Chapter 7: The 2nd Easiest Way to Quit

The Dream

I was a bit nervous the first time I recommended to a class of smokers "the absolutely easiest way to quit smoking" was to *stop doing smokes, just be who you already are.* After all, on the surface it's almost *too* easy, too obvious, and might even seem a bit insulting. (*I know I have to stop doing smokes! That's why I came here. But how do I stop doing smokes?*)

I introduced *the easiest way to quit* during the first class of folks who had signed up for our normal six session program. I told them that in the first class we would start with this "absolutely easiest way," and then in the second session move to the second easiest way, and then the third, and then the fourth and so on. For stop smoking classes across the country the average drop-out rate is close to fifty percent from the first class to the next. I was worried that what some might consider to be my "airy-fairy" recommendation for the easiest way to quit smoking might lead to a 100% drop out rate.

Nevertheless, in that first class we laughed and seemed to have a good time. "This certainly isn't what I was expecting," was the general response. The "easiest way" to quit smoking, for most smokers, seems almost too easy. (*There's nothing to do*!) Most smokers want to be told of something they can *do* to quit smoking. To be told they don't need to *do* anything, that they can be slackers, and/or just be their natural, ordinary selves seems, well, *too hard*!

The night before the second class was to meet, I had a dream. In the dream I was talking to a small group of people—my stop smoking class. I said, "Since there are so few of us, we can experiment with this new strategy. The strategy is **radical acceptance**." In that moment, after the words were spoken, I woke up.

The meaning of "radical acceptance" was so clear and obvious to me lying there in bed that at first I thought I didn't need to write it down. (Yea right.) Nevertheless, I got up in the dark in the middle of the night and wrote down those two words: *radical acceptance*.

As the dream was occurring the meaning of those two words was very clear. And in the morning, the meaning was still very clear. Here it is:

If we are going to *stop doing* and *just be* our natural selves for a brief moment, we must *accept everything* --- absolutely *everything* --- that rises up in our ordinary being in that moment. The word "radical" comes from the Latin word meaning "root." We accept ourselves – accept our ordinary being, and whatever is arising in it in that moment -- *down to the roots*. This is radical acceptance.

Radical acceptance is *not doing* anything to try to change whatever is arising in us in the moment. We allow ourselves to *just be* with whatever is arising. This is, obviously, completely contrary to what most of us have been taught most of our lives. (Thus, "radical" might also imply subversive!)

Most of us, especially if we're smokers, assume we have to *be* something or somebody different than what we are in this moment, who we are in this moment. Here's the basic argument I hear time and again against employing this "radical acceptance" strategy:

"I *can't* accept myself for who I am in this moment—I can't accept whatever is rising up in my being, because who *I am* is a smoker! If I accept who I am, and stop trying to *do* anything about it, I'll just continue to smoke for the rest of my life."

On the surface, it seems a reasonable argument. And yet...

A national Gallup Survey, reported in *American Health Magazine* found that people most often change their behaviors *not* because they are feeling bad or guilty about what they are doing or because of health issues or social pressure. Rather, **people most often change their behaviors when they are *feeling good about themselves* and want to feel still better**.

Radical acceptance—simply accepting who we are, accepting what is rising in our being in this moment --- is how we learn to be friendly with ourselves once again. As we did when we were kids. In other words, *radical acceptance is how we cease beating up on ourselves*!

In radical acceptance we neither exaggerate nor diminish what is rising up in us in this moment. We don't resist it or encourage it. We simply *be* with it. (This is, after all, who we are *being* in this moment!) We soon learn—observe—that whatever appears also disappears!

As we learn to accept, and simply *be with* who we are in this moment --- neither resist nor exaggerate the thoughts, feelings, sensations that are arising in our being in this moment – the inner struggles begin to diminish. The "divided mind," the two minds, start to harmonize.

This "radical acceptance" of who we are in this moment is not a part time job. It's not just something we do around our smoking. We are here learning to be at ease with ourselves, enjoy ourselves more throughout our whole day. Again, we're bringing peace —a moment at a time -- to the inner warfare. Here's why (it's worth repeating): **people most often change their behaviors when they are *feeling good about themselves* and want to feel still better,** rather than because of social pressures or health concerns.

Naturally, "radical acceptance" is easiest when we are feeling completely healthy, lying on a beach in Hawaii with the sun going down and our beautiful lover lying next to us and with the proceeds of our recent million dollar deal resting comfortably in our bank account.

It's quite easy to accept such moments. What rises up in our being is quite acceptable.

When we're stuck in Monday morning traffic, late for an appointment with our supervisor, having just had a fight with our spouse and our hemorrhoids are flaring up, accepting what rises up in *this* moment is not quite so easy. Nevertheless, the process is exactly the same: for a brief moment, we don't fight ourselves (or the traffic, or the time, or the spouse or the aching being). **We allow ourselves to be who we are in this moment.** What rises up in this moment will soon pass, just as what rose up on the beach in Hawaii passed. We can be friends with ourselves no matter where we are, or what state we're in.

Okay, relative to smoking: the thought rises up in our being, *"I'd really like to have a smoke."* If we've been trying to quit, wanting to quit, we might think, "Oh-oh, that's not a good thought, not a good urge. I shouldn't think that, shouldn't feel that." (Implying, "what can I do to stop thinking this, stop feeling this?")

But *this* is the thought, the urge that rose up in our ordinary being in that moment. With radical acceptance, we agree to cease fighting ourselves, cease fighting what rises up in our being. We accept the thought, the urge, "I'd really like to have a smoke." This doesn't mean we either act on the thought or prevent ourselves from acting on the thought. Rather, we simply don't give it energy one way or another. We simply *be with it*, accept it for what it is.

"But I'm really trying to quit," might be the next thought that rises up. So be it. We don't give this thought any energy either. We simply *be* with it, because it's what rose up in our being in that moment.

Here in the early stages, sometimes we might smoke, sometimes not—again, we simply *be* with whatever thought, feeling, sensation or action that happens to be present in this moment. (See how subversive this approach can get?)

So with what we've been looking at in the past couple of chapters, let's revisit and upgrade your first two homework assignments. To do that, though, we'll need another chapter.

[Note: The Back of the Bus discussion for this chapter will be found on page **231**.]

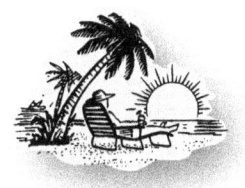

Chapter 8

Checking Your Homework

A baseball swing is a very finely tuned instrument. It is repetition, and more repetition, then a little more after that. ---- Reggie Jackson

Okay, we're back on the bus. Look around. Who's here, who's not?

For some readers, these last few chapters – where we pointed to radical acceptance and the absolutely easiest way to quit smoking --- did the trick, made things click. For these folks those chapters took them right to the Easy Exit Off Ramp. Seeing how close and easy the exit is, they found themselves naturally taking the exit. (For some it might have been after second or third or fourth reading of the entire book!)

So with those first observations, first chapters, some folks simply gave themselves permission to leave Smoke City the easy way. (Again, to summarize the observations: *You don't need to **do** anything. Just be who you already are.*)

So some of our fellow travelers are no longer here on the bus with us. They *stopped doing* their smokes and hopped off at the last stop, so to speak! No need to continue the tour. So be it. Let's be happy for them and wish them well.

Other readers may have likewise given themselves permission to *stop doing* their smokes but are nevertheless still riding along. They want the full tour. That's fine. They've paid their dues. We're happy to still have them along.

You yourself may decide: *if it's that easy, I might as well go ahead and do it*. Or more precisely, go ahead and *not* do it, *not* do the smokes. Just be yourself and let the chips fall where they may. Just accept yourself ---- accept whatever rises up --- when *not doing* your smokes. Allow yourself to be a slacker when it comes to *doing* smokes. It really can be that simple.

But quitting smoking --- *not doing* your smokes --- was *not* your homework. If you're still smoking, don't worry. Your stop is coming up, I guarantee. You'll recognize it when you see it. Again, your homework was *not* to stop smoking, though you're free to do that whenever the notion strikes you. And it *will* strike you, easily, naturally. In the meantime you don't need to *do* anything, except of course to keep doing your homework, which is to enjoy your life and observe.

Chapter 8: Checking Homework

In the next chapter you'll get a third homework assignment, but don't worry. The third homework assignment is even easier than the first two. But before we get to the new homework, let's check your old homework, make sure you're up to date.

As you know the first homework was to just be who you already are and enjoy your smokes. I trust you've been doing that. If you've already stopped *doing* your smokes --- but are still on the bus here with us, your homework now is to be yourself and enjoy *not doing* smokes, a moment at a time!

With what we've pointed out here I suspect you may now recognize how to be yourself and enjoy your smokes (and not smoking) at a deeper level, e.g., by simply -- and radically -- *accepting* who you are in this moment, whoever you happen to be. You enjoy by not beating yourself up, by letting whatever thoughts, feelings, sensations and actions that rise up in your being simply rise up, then fall away again. **Let yourself be who you are, right now, in this moment.** That's how you be yourself, and that's how you enjoy.

In the 1970's many of us were inspired by a classic little book written by Barry Stevens entitled *Don't Push the River, It Flows by Itself.* (The title neatly summarizes her insights.)

Relative to smoking, we don't need to push or pull the river of thoughts, feelings, sensations or actions that rise up and fall away each moment. They flow by themselves. Simply letting them flow is one way to enjoy our smokes more, though of course, we have to be brave to not beat up on ourselves for smoking.

And regarding beating yourself up --- feeling guilty, frustrated, ashamed about smoking --- here's a tip: If you find yourself still beating yourself up about your smokes, try to *enjoy* beating yourself up! It's understandable that such a counter-productive habit continues. If you're like most smokers you've probably been beating yourself up about it --- feeling guilty, frustrated, and ashamed --- for a long, long time. The stressing out, "beating up" habit is deeply engrained. So be it. Flow with it.

It doesn't help to beat yourself up about beating yourself up! **It doesn't help to stress out about stressing out!**

So just be with it. Homework number one is to be yourself and enjoy your smokes (and/or enjoy not smoking.) If part of your smoking routine was to beat yourself up about it, then enjoy that, too. *Radical acceptanc*e means accepting *everything* about ourselves that's rising up in this moment.

But let's keep it simple. Simply continue to enjoy yourself when you're smoking, and enjoy yourself when you're not smoking. Easy enough?

Homework number two, as you will remember, was to simply *observe*, or *look*. What we are observing is whatever is rising up in our being in this moment --- observing our thoughts, feelings, sensations and actions. I trust that these last two chapters have also taken this homework to a deeper level.

Most of us tend to *fight* with whatever's rising up in our being at any given moment; we tend to *fight* with what we are experiencing. (We can *observe* this tendency!) We tend to push (and pull) the river. We do this because we've been taught that for our own good—for our own well-being--- we need to *do* more of some things and *do* less of other things. At the mental level we've been taught we should hold on to our positive thoughts and feelings and get rid of our negative thoughts and feelings. Our well-being, we've been taught, depends on this inner and outer struggle between positive and negative.

In the meantime, we have a gazillion *neutral* thoughts, feelings and obligations --- it's time to take out the trash, do the dishes, get to the laundry, go to the store or watch our favorite television program. On the other hand it's also time to save the starving children, stop the wars, redeem the poor. All of this takes a lot of energy.

Our homework, though, is to simply *observe.* This doesn't mean we don't *do* the dishes, the laundry, the smokes. It doesn't mean we don't continue to feed the starving children.

But our homework is to simply *observe*. So what do we see?

We see what's rising up here in this moment. *Here I am, doing the dishes. Here I am doing the taxes, or reading this book. Here I am doing my smokes.* This simple homework is intended to take the pressure off. We don't have to *do* anything about what we observe, or about our thoughts, feelings, sensations or actions. **Our homework is to "just look," just observe, which is another way of saying, "*just be*" with whatever we see**, here in the moment, inside or out. (In some traditions this is called the "witness position," or witness consciousness. We don't need to worry whether we are fitting or not fitting into the traditions. We can *just observe*).

Yes of course, if we look and see a little old lady struggling to cross the street, we spontaneously reach out, offer an arm. Or when a can of beans starts to fall from the shelf we spontaneously reach to catch it. The homework, *"just observe"* doesn't mean we stop *doing* whatever needs to be done in the moment.

Rather, it helps us not to be so incessantly caught up in *doing, doing, doing,* so incessantly caught up in our thoughts that we forget our *being,* that we forget to simply observe (and maybe even *enjoy*) our ordinary lives as they are in this moment.

Relative to smoking, you may have noticed that most smokers are unconsciously caught up in *doing-doing- doing* their smokes.

When, in the other areas of our lives, we consciously take the emphasis off of all our *doing* and put it on our momentary *seeing*, or *being*, we spontaneously and effortlessly start to loosen the habit of *doing-doing* smokes. So not only relative to smoking, but in all areas of your life, allow yourself to simply look at, be with, what is arising in the moment. Such looking takes the pressure off. You don't need to either push or pull the river (of being) that is flowing in and around you in this moment. You'll act— you'll *do*--- just fine without all the fuss.

But again, let's not make it too complicated. For now, continue to just be yourself and enjoy, and observe. We want to make this journey effortless.

Homework number one: be yourself and enjoy your smokes (and/or enjoy not smoking.)

Homework number two: Observe. (Just look at, be with, who you already are in this moment.) Easy, yes? Okay. You're ready for your third homework assignment.

[Note: The Back of the Bus discussion for this chapter will be found on page **236**.]

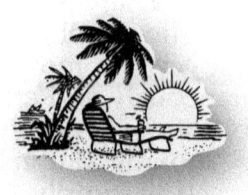

Chapter 9
Homework Assignment Three:
More Little *Ahh* Moments!

Enjoy the little things, for one day you may look back and realize they were the big things.
-- Robert Brault

Okay, here's easy homework assignment number three: Consciously, intentionally, give yourself more little *ahh* moments every day. Remember *ahh* moments?

To refresh: We isolated that brief moment after we haven't been able to smoke, or have been denying ourselves a smoke, and then we finally cave in, or get to where we finally are free to smoke. We take that first big inhale and then exhale, *ahh*... That's an *ahh* moment. Every smoker knows this delicious, brief, totally satisfied *ahh* moment.

In that brief moment, if you will notice, you are content to be right where you are, doing what you're doing. You are experiencing *radical acceptance* of who you are and what you are doing, feeling experiencing in that moment. You are happy to *just be* who you already are in that brief moment.

Yes, of course, by the third or fourth inhale or exhale, or sooner --- in the next moment or two --- we often start to beat ourselves up again or get lost again in *doing* this, that or something else so the *ahh* moment, the *ahh* relief, the radical acceptance, begins to fade. So sooner or later we light up another one, hoping for another *ahh* moment, for more radical acceptance.

Here's a profound little secret: **We don't need the first puff of a long-sought cigarette to give ourselves these little *ahh* moments** --- to be content right where we are, doing what we're doing. We don't need a smoke to experience *radical acceptance* of ourselves and our circumstance.

As we observed, contrary to general belief it is *not* the physical nicotine that gives us this *ahh* moment. We're not getting enough nicotine from one puff to bring such relief. The relief comes from our mental and emotional shift from *doing, doing, doing* to *just being*. For just a moment we allow ourselves to *just be* right where we are, *accept* right where we are. **The *ahh* moment is relief from wanting to be somewhere other than where we are**, e.g., relief from *not accepting* where we are and what we are doing!

Again, we can observe that the *ahh* moment doesn't last very long. Often by the third or fourth puff or even sooner we're thinking about something else, or reading a magazine or drinking our coffee. This *ahh* moment of radical acceptance is very brief.

So here's the homework: Every day start giving yourself more and more of these brief *ahh* moments --- where you take your attention off of *doing, doing, doing* and, just for a moment, allow yourself to simply **enjoy being right where you are, doing what you're doing, however mundane it might be.**

Ahh, I'm walking into work again. *Ahh*, I'm doing the dishes. *Ahh*, studying the blueberries in the grocery store.

Yes, we can still be aware of the *ahh* moments that occasionally arise with our smokes, but the homework is to give ourselves these *ahh* moments without the smokes. And they don't have to be huge, earth shattering, sky-opening moments of rejoicing. Let them be simple, small, easy. We might even call them "baby *ahhs*."

More examples: we wake in the morning. *Ahh*, sunshine from a new day. Or even before the sunshine, *ahh*, these warm covers. When we're in our morning shower, *ahh*, warm water. And then at breakfast, *ahh*, oatmeal. On the drive to work, *ahh*, made that green light.

To be absolutely clear about this homework, let's look again at the *"ahh"* experience from the first puff, the first inhale and exhale of a long-awaited smoke. It's *ahh* because we are happy to *simply be* right there, in that moment, doing what we're doing, feeling what we're feeling. We're not fighting ourselves. We're *accepting* ourselves and the moment. We're not trying to be anywhere else!

Again, we can observe: It's not a huge *ahh*, like *"ahh, I won the lotto,"* or *"ahh, I won the Nobel Prize,"* or *"ahh, I made it to the top of Mt. Everest."* The *ahh* we get from the first drag of a smoke is much simpler, more mundane, more ordinary. Your homework is to be brave enough to consciously give yourself more *ahh's* during the day. *Ahh*, warm toast and butter.

Why this homework works to decrease smoking:

Let's imagine that you've just smoked five cigs in a row, without thinking much about it. No, let's make it ten. You've just smoked half a pack, maybe sitting with an old friend, drinking beer or worrying about the mortgage, whatever. You've just smoked half a pack. No let's make it three quarters of a pack. Whatever it takes, you've just saturated yourself with smokes. Lots of smokes, in a very short while. Rather than *ahh*, you feel *uggh*. We've all been there, yes? When we've smoked too much?. *Uggh*.

We walk out into fresh night air, say goodbye to our friend, start to walk back to our car and as we do, out of habit, we reach for another smoke. We suddenly recognize what we're doing, and our hand stops. We put the smokes back in our pocket. *Uggh. I don't need another smoke.*

It's very easy to *not* smoke in that circumstance, yes? We're already filled up. We're already full. We've smoked our brains out. We don't need any more. It's like putting gas in the tank. When it's full, it's full. An invisible little switch goes off that says, "That's enough."

Wouldn't it be nice to feel this way about our smokes all the time? "No thanks. Don't need another one. I've had enough." We're not holding ourselves back. We're not being disciplined, white-knuckling it. **We simply don't need another one**.

For many long term smokers --- you may be one of them --- it's not only a particular moment where they have smoked enough. They have come to a *season* in their lives where they realize that over the years they've smoked enough. For these folks, they discover it's fairly easy to quit smoking simply because in their lives *they've smoked enough already, thanks.*

I remember one old geezer in one of my classes (I can call him a geezer because I'm fast becoming a geezer too) who had quit on the first or second night. After four or five weeks someone asked him if he didn't feel tempted to fall back, to start smoking again.

"The idea comes up," he admitted. "But after smoking for fifty-five years, I already know what it's like. Been there, done that. Enough's enough."

When we are brave enough to allow ourselves more and more brief *ahh* moments during the day — when we start deeply *accepting* ourselves in various moments just as we are, right where we are, happy to be doing what we're doing --- we discover that this is what we're actually looking for in a smoke. When we give ourselves more and more *ahh* moments, the smokes themselves start to lose their importance, and thus start to lose their grip.

As we practice being at ease with where we are in this moment, deeply accepting, not fighting what we're doing --- **not wanting something different than what is right here, *radically accepting* ourselves and the moment** — our *wants* spontaneously grow lighter, more friendly, and then effortlessly begin to dissolve and flow away. Our "wants" will continue to come and go, rise and fall as long as we walk the earth. But **maturity comes when we directly experience that what we are looking for is the "*ahh*" itself**, the deep acceptance of life as it is appearing in this moment. (*Ahhh*....)

So that's homework assignment number three. Allow yourself more *ahh* moments, whenever you remember to do so throughout the day. Not only accept but even *enjoy* who you are, where you are, moment by moment. Easy, yes?

Let's be very clear about this assignment. It is *not* that you should stop doing your smokes and instead give yourself *ahh* moments. No. The homework is to simply give yourself more *ahh* moments, whether you're smoking or not!

Again, I recognize that this is not the approach that you will find in any other stop smoking program. (And again I remind you that most stop smoking programs have a seventy percent or greater failure rate.) I recognize that each of these three homework-assignments --- (1. Be yourself and enjoy your smokes; 2. observe; 3. give yourself more *ahh* moments) are different than what you were expecting, or what you've tried in the past.

The good news is that *all* of your homework here in the fifteen easy years approach is going to be this easy. You're going to discover that quitting smoking can be much easier, more natural, more familiar than you ever dreamed possible. (*ahh*...) Guaranteed.

Okay. We've finished this chapter, you have your homework. Back on the bus (*ahh*.) Where to next? How about the hospital, the nursing home and then the hospice center?

Chapter 9: More Ahh Moments

No? You don't want to go there? Sorry, we need a quick drive-by simply because this is the neighborhood where most smokers go when trying to quit smoking. I promise, we'll make it quick. Ready? *Ahh,* here we go…

[Note: The Back of the Bus discussion for this chapter will be found on page **237.**]

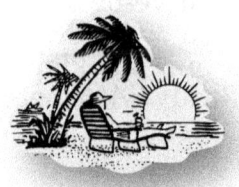

Chapter 10

The Hardest Way to Quit: Physical Health Concerns

Baseball is ninety percent mental and the other half is physical. —Yogi Berra

You have three easy homework assignments --- be yourself, enjoy, observe, *ahh*. And you've been shown the absolutely easiest way to quit smoking --- *just be*, and then accept whatever comes up in your being. This is the foundation of the easy way to quit smoking. Seems almost too easy, yes?

So okay, now let's take a look at the hard way, just because it's expected of us. To do this we need to drive our bus over to the hospital, and then by the old folks home, and finally over to hospice. Curiously, this neighborhood is where most smokers think they are supposed to *start* when getting ready to quit.

Chapter 10: The Hardest Way to Quit

When I ask a new class on the first evening why they each want to quit smoking, nine times out of ten the first answers come under the heading of "health reasons." Everybody has their own particular, personal health reason, of course, but most everybody in class is quick to agree that "health reasons" are the number one reasons for quitting. This is understandable.

Even young healthy people without dire diagnoses say they want to quit because they are worried about what putting smoke into their lungs all day every day is doing to their body. They can *feel* what it's doing, and it doesn't feel healthy.

Most older smokers have a direct personal experience of the adverse effects of smoking on their body, either brief or long term. And if they don't have such a direct personal experience, their doctors will warn them of the harmful effects, and the media will remind them, and their families will nag them with the information again and again and again.

And lest we forget (how can we?) even the Surgeon General now offers new warnings on absolutely every pack of cigarettes that these things are as addictive as heroin or cocaine, can cause fatal lung disease, cancer, strokes and heart disease, can harm children both before and after they are born and that quitting smokes will greatly reduce risks to health. (Duh.)

It took twenty-five years but the cig packs now finally carry all the warnings that most smokers were carrying around in their head. The advent of more graphic and detailed health warnings on cigarettes was undoubtedly inevitable, and will prove useful and necessary in helping smokers quit, or, more directly, in dissuading young kids from repeating their experiments with the noxious weed. That's a good thing.

I'm obviously not arguing here against the centuries of data documenting the health hazards of smoking. Yes, *centuries*! As far back as 1604 King James was one of the many early voices pointing out the health hazards of smoking. Other authoritative voices have been offering such warnings in every country in every century since, though it's fashionable these days to pretend that when we were kids we didn't *really* know about the health hazards. Only in the last fifty years has the hard evidence against smoking begun to have a noticeable influence on the powerful economic and social momentum that the tobacco industry has enjoyed. (Yes, granted, as kids they still had "smoking rooms" set aside in the hospitals. My own high school offered us a dedicated smoking area right outside the gym.)

In the last one hundred years the health hazards of tobacco have been meticulously and repeatedly demonstrated in literally thousands of scientific studies offering irrefutable

Chapter 10: The Hardest Way to Quit

statistics. We all know that smoking is not good for our physical health. No debate there. And yet...

Here are two more curious facts about the dangers of smoking that don't get a lot of public attention:

1. **Most smokers are *already* very much aware of the health risks of smoking. In fact, research suggests that most smokers gauge the risks from smoking as *higher* than do non-smokers!**
2. **Although smokers gauge the risks from smoking as higher than do non-smokers, most smokers also privately assume that they themselves will somehow more likely be able to *dodge* these long term harmful effects.**

Obviously, health concerns have motivated millions of smokers to quit. No argument.

"You want to quit smoking, I'll tell you how to quit," an old friend blurted out when he heard I was a stop smoking coach. "Just have a heart attack. Hear angel feathers. That's what happened to me. I went from three packs a day to zero, in an instant."

That's one way to do it, for some people. It has happened this way time and time again. And some people don't need anything as serious as a heart attack. Maybe just a slight case of bronchitis, or a bout with the flu, or sinus problems, and for some reason these small health problems, in that time, and in that place, are sufficient to bring these people to a point where they recognize they are something bigger than the smokes, and they can say, "that's it, I'm done."

On the other hand, many others are like my construction worker client --- now out of work because of health reasons --- who confessed to me, "You know, I've already had three heart attacks. You'd think I'd learn my lesson. But I still can't kick these stupid things."

People waiting for organ transplants have to be smoke free for at least six months, and in some cases (like for a new heart) have to be smoke-free for a year before they even get put on the waiting list! This is not just anti-tobacco prejudice. It's based on real life case histories. Doctors were dumfounded that ex-smokers who had been given a new heart would, six to eight months after a successful operation, start smoking again! (I had one client who was quitting in order to be put on to the "heart transplant" list. She told me, "One year after I get my new heart, I'm going to start smoking again." What?)

One of the saddest and most baffling cases I've worked with was a dear little old lady who at one time had been given the diagnosis of lung cancer, the big bogeyman for every smoker. She went through many operations and chemo treatments and actually succeeded in reversing the diagnosis. The docs had pronounced that her lungs were clear.

Alas, she started smoking again. And then, a year or so later, the docs found spots on her lungs again, and scheduled her to come in for more chemo treatments. The last time she was in my office --- on a Monday morning --- she told me, "Well, I don't start chemo until Thursday, so maybe I'll make Wednesday night my quit date." Wednesday night? What?

A history of the disease, new spots on the lungs and chemo on Thursday! If facing immediate health hazards --- immediate prospect of death! --- were a sufficient motivator, one would assume she had hit the jackpot in regards to health hazard motivation. But my little old lady friend figured she could wait until Wednesday night. (The dear woman suffered complications with the chemo, ended up in the hospital and passed away that weekend.)

Yes, of course, many people immediately quit when they hear a dire diagnosis. Ten years after the landmark 1964 Surgeon General's report on the hazards of smoking, coupled with increased cigarette taxes and education programs, the smoking rates in the U.S. had dropped by nearly forty percent. In the last ten years, however, the decrease in smoking has radically slowed and in some areas for some populations started to climb back up. Fear of health hazards--- fear of imminent death itself---appears to be an inefficient motivator. Haven't we all known friends or relatives forced to live with oxygen tubes strapped to their noses who still smoke? Why?

Quite simply, and easily, in spite of the statistics pointing to the dangers of smoking, none of us ever actually experience ourselves as a *statistic*. On the contrary. We each experience ourselves as a living presence, somewhat magical, clearly multi-dimensional and often mysterious. Yes, of course we want to do what's healthy for us and stay away from what's not healthy. And we're pretty good at it, most of the time. Most of us don't sniff airplane glue or drive 95 miles an hour without a seat belt or go ice climbing in our tennis shoes.

Although there are exceptions, and seasons and reasons for those exceptions, most of us don't focus our lives --- narrow our lives --- to the single pursuit of physical health. We generally have so much more *happening* right now in our lives--- money, work, family relationships, household demands, social and political uncertainties, television, the movies, the internet, the dog needs walking and barbarians are at the door --- that health concerns are ordinarily just one small band of color in a whole rainbow of concerns.

Of course, when health starts to fail or when we have a sudden problem, then our health suddenly or gradually becomes a larger and larger concern. Still, smoking itself becomes just one band of color --- maybe a flashing red --- in the entire rainbow.

Curiously, I've had many, many clients whose primary life focus has indeed been on their health issues --- chronic pain, a severe disease diagnosis, even COPD or emphysema --- who still consider their smoking as a small, tangential irritant in the larger challenge.

The problem with "health concerns" as a motivator for quitting smoking --- as politically correct as such concerns may be --- is that this approach relies on the immediate presence of sickness and death, or near death, or the fear of sickness and death to get us moving. And when we are sick or near death, or deeply frightened, we generally aren't thinking clearly, aren't happy doing what we are doing, not at peace, or at ease with where we are. **Whatever decisions we make in this state are generally quite weak and fleeting.**

So it will be useful here to again remember the Gallup survey which found **that people most often change their behaviors because they are feeling *good* about themselves and want to feel still better rather than because of social pressure or health concerns.**

And it might also be useful to remember what Plato observed: "Attention to health is life's greatest hindrance." Plato's view may be a somewhat silly, even extreme position, and yet...

"The doctor told me I need to quit smoking or I'll die, " a long-term, handyman client told me when he once again came in for more nicotine patches, which he thought should be the solution to his two-pack-a-day problem. (For many years in a row he would come to get patches until his "quota" had run out--- and we have a very high quota. We are willing to work with people for six months or more. When my friend's quota had run out, or he saw that patches alone were not doing the trick, I wouldn't see him for a while. Then six months or a year or two later he'd show back up, telling me, "I'm really going to do it this time," his faith in the patches deeply intact, in spite of their past performances.)

"The doctor told me I need to quit smoking or I'll die," the handyman told me, again.

"Jim," I said (not his real name) "How long ago did the doctor tell you that?"

He grinned, shook his head, a little ashamed. He knew that I knew. "I know, I know. It's been what, three and half, four years now? I guess the doctor didn't know what he was talking about, huh? " And then Jim went into another coughing spell. I handed him a glass of water.

The grim joke in the smoking business: "Well, they took out my left lung, but I still have my right one. Got a light?"

Chapter 10: The Hardest Way to Quit

Again, our concerns about health are quite rational, deeply documented, personally and politically correct reasons for quitting. And millions of smokers have quit for such reasons. And many are quite happy and at peace with their new non-smoking. Others are the ones who confess, "I quit smoking five years ago, and have wanted a smoke every day since!" Or who, five or ten years after quitting, run into some life problems that lead them back to finally give in to temptation and return to smoking.

Although health reasons are good reasons for quitting and *should* be good enough reasons, they often are not *sufficient* reasons. To use "physical health reasons" as our reason to quit smoking means we might actually wait until we are physically so sick in bed that we can't lift our arms, can't lift our head from the pillow. *Then* it will be physically impossible to smoke so *then* we'll stop smoking, at least for a while. Until we recover, and are physically able to do it again.

Let's look again closely, with fresh eyes at what it *really* means to quit for health reasons. At the physical level, as I just pointed out, we can actually continue to smoke until we are physically confined to bed unable to lift our head or lift our hands. Or we can continue to smoke until our lungs are so congested that we can't physically inhale the smoke.

So unless and until we are in these very dire physical straights --- where we literally are too *physically* sick to smoke --- **when we say we are going to quit for "physical health reasons" we are in fact relying on our *mental* reasons.**

We are *thinking* about how physically sick we are or have been or might be. We are trying to use our *thinking* about bad health or good health as a way to quit. When we are worried about our health we are making mental projections based on fear, loss and shame. None of us like to mentally dwell on such projections. So we turn our attention elsewhere. "I know I should quit, I've been coughing a lot, but first I need to do the laundry."

To use "health reasons" as a way to quit smoking means we have to train ourselves to keep thinking about our health, either good health or bad health, all day every day until we're done with the smokes. Very few of us are so mentally disciplined that we can keep our attention focused on a single topic all day every day, especially a topic that we don't enjoy. Nevertheless, this is the way many, many smokers approach quitting. Indeed, smokers are encouraged to approach quitting in this way. "Just think how good you'll feel. Remember how bad you felt."

Yes, we can do this, for a moment or two. And then repeat it again, for a moment or two. To ask us to do this all day every day, **instead of smoking**, which we do all day every day without thinking, is asking a great deal. No wonder the success rates for quitting are so low.

Again, of course we *can* use our worries, and/or the daily evidence of health problems as a motivator to *stop doing* our smokes. Many smokers have. And "health reasons" are the traditional motivators behind *not doing* smokes. But let's be honest with ourselves: quitting for health reasons, although politically correct, is in fact the hardest way of doing it. Hasn't this been our experience, over many, many years?

Enough said. Let's get back to the easy ways of quitting, okay?

In the next chapter we'll look at how smoking --- *doing* our *s*mokes --- is not only an action, but obviously a lifestyle. We'll look at how *not doing* smokes can itself simply be an easy, obvious lifestyle that we are inspired to easily, gently adopt over days and weeks. *Not doing* smokes as a lifestyle choice?

Back on the bus…

[Note: The Back of the Bus discussion for this chapter will be found on page **241.**]

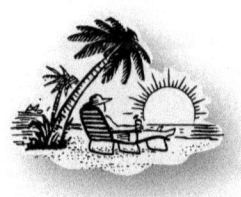

Chapter 11
Invitation to a (Momentary) Lifestyle

"My definition of success is to live your life in a way that causes you to feel a ton of pleasure and very little pain --- and because of your lifestyle, have the people around you feel a lot more pleasure than they do pain." --- Anthony Robbins

Okay, we're back on the bus, heading across town to your old neighborhood, where you lived when you first started smoking. My pleasant job is to help you find your way to the Easy Exit Off Ramp. To do so, I'd like to point out a few things about your old stomping grounds (smoking grounds?) that you may have forgotten, or maybe didn't even notice when you lived there.

First, according to the National Drug Survey, and as you probably already know, ninety percent of all smokers started smoking at age eighteen or before. And fifty percent of

Chapter 11: A momentary Lifestyle

these started at age fifteen or before. So chances are, you started smoking fairly young. Smoking is a "lifestyle" that most of us picked up --- starting with a few quick moments -- when we were still kids.

In my first meeting with new clients I generally ask how old they were when they first smoked. When they tell me, I then ask (as a joke), "Did someone have a gun to your head?"

Alas, one young man answered, "Well, yes, in a way. I started smoking when I was a soldier in Iraq." I've had others answer that they started smoking in response to some violent threat or circumstance. One size does not fit all.

Nevertheless, for most of us, the answer is no, of course not, nobody had a gun to our head. We did it as a goof, trying to be cool, trying to grow up, wanting to be in with the in-crowd. For most of us, our parents were smokers, or our siblings, or a close relative or good friend. Smoking was a "lifestyle" that most of us were introduced to by people we loved, or admired, wanted to emulate. Smoking was a lifestyle that many around us, when we were kids, had already adopted.

Since we were just kids **it was totally natural for us to emulate the lifestyle of the people around us,** just as both Aboriginal kids and Jet-set kids naturally adopt the lifestyle of the people around them. Nevertheless, many folks have told me, "I started because of peer pressure."

I suggest no, it wasn't really peer *pressure*. It was peer *adventure*. That's what we kids were doing. Again, for most of us, nobody had a gun to our head. We were just having fun, hanging out with friends, having an adventure, wanting to grow up. For just a moment we wanted to try out the "lifestyle" of cool people. Or rebel people. Brave people. After we tried out this lifestyle for the first time, (after we smoked for the first time) we tried it again, and then again. One moment after another, one circumstance after another, until we had we made this new lifestyle our own.

I titled my first stop smoking book *The Enlightened Smoker's Guide to Quitting* because for most of us when we first start smoking we're hoping to be somebody new on earth, somebody more real, somebody more cool, e.g., we were looking for enlightenment. We didn't know this is what we we're doing --- looking for enlightenment, or a new lifestyle, a new *persona*--- but isn't that what kids do, testing life, **responding to life, willing to have new life adventures? The basic urge—to grow, to change, to explore --- is actually very healthy!**

And it worked, a little bit. Smoking did in fact make us feel like somebody new, and maybe even a little more real, a little more cool, more grown up, if just a little bit. It was a great adventure, learning this new lifestyle. The *effects* of smoking were not that great. But learning the smoking *lifestyle* was new, fun, enjoyable! So be it. (If we hadn't experienced that lifestyle as fun, enjoyable, we wouldn't have continued with it. Many of our friends tried out the smoking lifestyle and didn't enjoy it. Those who didn't enjoy the lifestyle quickly gave it up!)

So here's the key: *Not doing* **smokes can be understood simply as learning how to adopt a fun new** *lifestyle*!

Although we didn't use these words, isn't this what we were doing when we first fell into smoking? And just as when we first started smoking the physical effects felt a bit strange and disorienting (and fun!) --- that's part of why we did I --- so too the physical effects of *not doing* smokes may appear a bit strange and disorienting and fun, if we let them be! In both cases--- starting smoking and ending smoking--- it's the excitement of a new *lifestyle* that keeps you going down that street!

In other words, we can use the same ramp to get *out* of Smoke City that we used to get in! We can allow ourselves to remember the courage, the fun, the adventurous attitude that we had when we were kids as we secretly tried out a new lifestyle, wanting to be cool, to fit in.

Here in our maturity we discover that by *not doing* our smokes we are again secretly trying out a very *cool*, hip, even enlightened lifestyle! It's never too late to learn to adopt a new lifestyle, just as, when we were kids, we didn't feel it was too early!

Allen Carr, the bestselling author of *Alan Carr's Easy Way to Quit Smoking*, was a five pack-a-day smoker. (You have to work at that --- reach for a smoke before you get out of bed, and then light your new one using the hot tip of the old one.) When Carr finally quit smoking he said he found it was fairly easy. Although he wrote many books about the easy way, and created a five hour workshop to present the easy way, in his books he boils it down to two sentences:

1. Make the decision you're never going to smoke again; and

2. Don't mope about it. Rejoice!

I don't know if Carr realized how powerful that second piece of advice really is. I often ask my clients, "When you started smoking, did you mope about it?" They generally grin, chuckle. No, of course not.

Again, **let's use the same gate to get <u>out</u> of smoking that we used to get in**. We can allow ourselves to make the *momentary <u>not-doing</u>* of smokes as much fun, as much of an adventure as we once made the *momentary doing*. Can it be this easy? How do we *do* that? We *do* that simply by *not moping* about it, accepting ourselves just as we are, and then let *not-doing* smokes be a fun new lifestyle!

A lifestyle? Again, smoking is something that we *do*. Not smoking is something we *cease* doing.

Chapter 11: A momentary Lifestyle

We can observe that lifestyles are often adopted by choosing *not to do* particular actions. For example:

The vegetarian lifestyle is a lifestyle of *not doing* meat! Some folks choose a lifestyle of *not doing* television. Others choose not to swear, or not to covet, not to drink, not to vote Republican or not to vote Democrat (or just not to vote!).

Of course, we can also choose a lifestyle based on what we *do* --- say, casual sex with strangers or drinking every night (sometimes these two lifestyles go together!) Or wearing robes and chanting mantras or running five miles every morning.

Still, *not doing* smokes can be seen simply as a chosen lifestyle. A lifestyle we *enjoy*! Obviously, you are not quitting smokes because you want to be miserable. (Nor did you *start* smoking because you wanted to be miserable.) No, you're quitting --- *not doing* the smokes-- for the same reason you started the smokes: because you want to have more fun, want to enjoy your life more. Yes?

So how do we do that? We've already covered this ground. Here's the basic "Enjoy Life" lifestyle practice that I share with most of my clients.

The Basic *Enjoy Life* Lifestyle Principle:

Enjoying our lives is the healthiest, most natural and most loving thing we can do for ourselves and all those around us.

Observation 1: *We only enjoy our lives for brief moments at a time.*

Observation 2: *We forget to enjoy our lives when we get caught up with what we are "doing" in the moment (through thoughts, feelings or actions) rather than with simply being in the moment.*

The Lifestyle Practice: **To enjoy our lives more, we take the emphasis off of whatever we are *doing* in the moment and simply remember again to *enjoy being* in the moment, no matter what we happen to be *doing*.**

We repeat this simple practice of *enjoying being here in this moment* – regardless of what thoughts, feelings, sensations or actions are arising in this moment. We adopt this lifestyle simply by *enjoying being here in this moment* whenever we remember to do it, wherever we happen to be.[1] *Ahh*, Walmart again.

This is our new lifestyle. We are learning to simply enjoy our lives more, a moment at a time, regardless of what we are doing or what is happening. Enjoying our lives does not depend on what we are *doing*. It doesn't depend on what we are thinking. It doesn't depend on what we are feeling. It depends only on taking

---

[1] Thanks, a tip of the hat and a deep bow to Candice O'Denver and The Balanced View Community for inspiring earlier versions of this simple practice and Candice's brilliant book *One Simple Change Makes Life Easy*.

Chapter 11: A momentary Lifestyle

the emphasis off of *doing* and putting it onto *being* here in this moment. Therefore, anybody can take up this lifestyle at any time, regardless of their circumstance.

And if we look closely --- isn't this "lifestyle practice" what we are trying to do with our smokes, but not succeeding very well? When we stop for a smoke aren't we just trying to enjoy our lives more, for a brief moment or two, no matter what else we are doing? And when we are already enjoying our lives --- don't we in those moments *forget to* smoke?

Again, this simple, enjoyable lifestyle that we are learning to adopt is *not* a lifestyle based on something we have to *do* --- or based on something we have done or are hoping to do. So it's actually a much simpler, easier, more elegant lifestyle than the smoking lifestyle, where we are forced to *do* something all the time, or *get ready* to *do* something, or *do* something about what we just *did*. Rather, this new lifestyle is based simply on *enjoying being alive*, here in this very moment, regardless of what we are thinking, feeling, sensing or *doing*.

If you will remember, or observe, this is what kids do all the time. Most kids most of the time are enjoying their lives. They are simply enjoying *being*, until we teach them to focus on *doing*, until we *insist* that they focus on *doing*.

When we give ourselves permission to learn this new lifestyle—learn to take the emphasis off of *doing, doing, doing* and putting it simply onto *being* here in this moment, we get a taste of natural freedom. We discover we can *enjoy being* ourselves no matter what thoughts, feelings or sensations happen to be rising up in our being in that moment. When we learn to enjoy simply *being*, for brief moments throughout the day, we discover we are not so bound or driven by old urges, patterns and compulsions. We aren't fighting them, but we aren't driven by them either. Putting the emphasis on *being* rather than *doing* is the doorway to freedom.

It seems almost too simple, doesn't it? That we can walk away from smoking if we simply allow ourselves to *enjoy being* here in this moment? All of our training, and our cultural conditioning leads us to believe that that we must *do* something in order to quit smoking, just as we are trained we must *do, do, do* something special in order to enjoy our lives. I have discovered—as have my clients—that this is faulty training. We can enjoy our lives in *any* moment regardless of what we are doing, if we simply allow ourselves such enjoyment.

So relative to smoking, is there something we are supposed to *do* when we cease doing our smokes? No. We don't have to *do* anything. We simply enjoy the moment, no matter what thoughts, feelings or sensations are rising up and falling away. We cease fighting ourselves. In other words, we adopt a certain *radical acceptance* of our experiences in this moment. We live free of the struggles, the wars. *Ahh...*

Okay. Everybody back on the bus. Enjoy whatever reactions you might be having to this chapter. If you want to, you can use this "change of lifestyle" approach to go ahead and take the Easy Exit Off Ramp out of Smoke City --- simply *don't do* your smokes anymore. You already know everything you need to know. But no pressure here. Taking the Off Ramp is not your homework. We're just having a (hopefully excellent) adventure here.

Let's drive the bus a bit more around the old neighborhood, see if we can spot that young hitchhiker we knew from so many years ago. Let's just *enjoy being* in this moment... and the continuing ride, this unfolding adventure, here on this wondrous planet.

[Note: The Back of the Bus discussion for this chapter will be found on page **246.**]

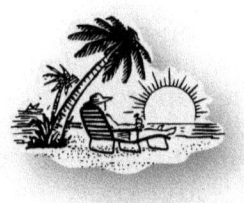

Chapter 12
Picking Up and Ditching Hitchhikers

"Perhaps it's impossible to wear an identity without becoming what you pretend to be."
— Orson Scott Card

Since the bus is still circling the old neighborhood, where you first picked up the smoking lifestyle, let's revisit how that happened, and put it into perspective. And then we'll drive around to where you now live, see what's changed over the years. Again, our plan is to use the same ramp to get out of smoking as we used to get in. So to look back at our experience when we first started and compare it to where we're living today will be useful for starting our new lifestyle, making our way out of Smoke City.

Chapter 12: The Hitchhiker

As we discussed in previous chapters, when we first started smoking we were simply trying to enjoy ourselves, trying to grow up, fit in, be cool. This wasn't an original or unique idea. We were following what we were taught, either overtly or covertly.

Again, most of us have been taught, from a very early age, that we have to *do* something in order to achieve some future well-being. So we're always looking for something to *do*, be it major or minor, in this moment or in this year, that will somehow improve our lives, that will lead to more well-being. (When we take a moment to observe, as we encouraged in the last chapter, we discover that our *being* is already quite well and full and whole, thank you very much, right where we are. Nevertheless, we've all been trained, here on planet earth, to *do, do, do,* running off to the horizon in search of something new. Welcome to the monkey fun house.)

Okay, let's circle the bus to the neighborhood you inhabited right *before* you started *doing* your smokes in your quest to achieve well-being. Whether you were in middle school or high school, (or earlier or later) you were simply living your life, doing what you were doing, trying to get along, probably not even thinking about whether to smoke or not smoke. **As kids, for most of us, the question of smoking or not smoking wasn't even on our radar**. (I've talked with many clients who said, *yes, it was* on their radar when they were young and they were vehemently *opposed* to it, generally because it was something their parents were doing, or something their parents warned against.)

For most of us, we were neither passionately for nor against smoking, in the same way we're neither for nor against Mongolian horse polo. (Smoking, of course, was much more prevalent in our culture than Mongolian horse polo, but still, most of us hadn't given smoking a lot of thought one way or the other before we took it up.)

Okay, so we were just living our lives, doing what we were doing as kids, or teens, or young adults, not thinking much about smoking or not smoking, and then it happened. The opportunity arose, and we took it.

To make it very clear, and so that we're all on the same page with our various smoking histories, let's use a metaphor. Let's pretend that the first opportunity to smoke happened this way: when you were younger, just for fun, and to have an adventure, maybe with your friends, you picked up a hitchhiker—we'll call him Mr. Tobacco --- who was standing beside the road. (He himself was pretending to be just a kid at the time.) You were a brave, fun-loving bunch, picking up hitchhikers was part of it. Ahh, youth!

Chapter 12: The Hitchhiker

Let's pretend you were the driver. Naturally, when the hitchhiker first hopped in you asked, *where you going?*

No where special, Mr. T., the hitchhiker replied. *Where are **you** going?*

"I'm just going to school," you said, or to work or to the party, or wherever you happened to be going at the time.

"That's fine. I'll just tag along," Mr. T. the hitchhiker said with a shrug and a grin. "Don't worry about me. I don't really have anywhere else to go."

So Mr. T. the hitchhiker tagged along, started hanging out. (Come to find out, he really *didn't* have anywhere else to go.) The good news was that he actually fit in quite well with you and your friends, maybe even with your family. Whether you were being serious or having fun, were stressed out or relaxing, Mr. T. the hitchhiker was right there, made no complaints, quietly hung in there with you. You became great friends. Such great friends, in fact, that over the next weeks and months, or maybe years, Mr. T. the hitchhiker slowly, quietly, unobtrusively moved in with you.

"We're going out to dinner," someone would say. Or on vacation, or off to work, or to the store.

"Great," Mr. T. the hitchhiker says, no matter where it is you're going. "I'll go with you."

"But I'm going to church," you say, or to the synagogue, or to grandpa and grandmas, where Mr. T. was certainly not invited.

"That's okay," he says, "Don't worry about me. I'll wait outside."

So it's been a number of years now. Maybe even a lot of years that Mr. T. the hitchhiker has been tagging along, no matter where you go. Even just staying home, Mr. T. is there. **You're so close now --- you've been together since you were kids --- that you think alike, feel the same things, wear the same clothes.** You and Mr. T. are so close you feel like you're joined at the hip, almost Siamese Twins, though in fact you're not.

You're so close that you've forgotten that this guy is a "pick up" friend that at one time you didn't even know, let alone think about continually. He's now as much a part of you as your telephone number, or street address. In fact, *closer* to you than your phone number or street address. Mr. T., is no longer the hitchhiker, but rather your bosom buddy.

Lately, however, he's starting to get on your nerves. It bugs you that Mr. T. steadily, quietly but insistently borrows money from you. *Every* day. Five bucks here, five bucks there, but it's real regular, and starting to add up. This guy doesn't work but he needs money all the time, even on weekends. And even though you yourself don't need to go to the store, Mr. T. the hitchhiker needs you to go to the store, so he can spend *your* five bucks. And he can't go there alone, so you take him.

And not only has Mr. T. the hitchhiker been borrowing money every day, he's also been quietly, almost unobtrusively borrowing other things from you. At first it was little things, like a new shirt or blouse or jacket that came back smelling funky, and sometimes even with a burn hole in it. The idiot. But you don't hear any apologies from him.

He's also been steadily borrowing little bits of your time-- five minutes here and five minutes there, but all day, every day. And the time he takes adds up, day after day, week after week, year after year. You see that Mr. T. takes up a *lot* of your time.

And hand in glove with time, Mr. T. the hitchhiker has been insistently asking for — and getting --- little bits of your *attention*. When you are doing something else, even late at night, Mr. T. the hitchhiker persistently calls to you, demanding just a bit more of your attention. You can put him off for a while, but when Mr. T. asks for your attention, sooner or later, you give it to him.

Because he has been borrowing your money, and your clothes, and your time and attention, and because other people know this is your relationship with Mr. T., your very own hitchhiker, you know that he has also borrowed some of your reputation, which he also brought back a little bit soiled. The idiot. Uggh.

And moving toward the last straw, as we drive this bus around your old neighborhood it's only fair to point out that Mr. T., the hitchhiker --- your old pal, your lifelong friend —has actually been quietly *stealing* from you. He's been stealing some of your most private, most treasured and almost irreplaceable possessions. Maybe you hadn't noticed his theft at first. But now you start to see that Mr. T. has been stealing, for his own use, your personal sense of smell. You don't have as much of it as you once did. And he's also been stealing your sense of taste. And finally, perhaps as *the* last straw, you realize Mr. T. the hitchhiker has been stealing for his own use larger and larger portions of your very *breath*! He's stealing what you use to *live with*! What you absolutely *need* to live with! Your *oxygen*!

"Give it back!" you shout.

But Mr. T. just shrugs, and turns away, as if he didn't hear you. He's not giving your oxygen back, at least not as long as he continues to live with you. It appears as though Mr.T. has no qualms, no guilt, no shame about stealing your oxygen, your very life, even if you don't have any oxygen to spare! (You might have to start buying extra oxygen! Or maybe you already are!) What kind of friend is this?

Chapter 12: The Hitchhiker

So you've come to the point (or you wouldn't be reading this book) where enough is enough. What you need to do is obvious. The question now is, how to evict Mr. T., this hitchhiker? How do you get this thief, this ex-old friend, this stranger/hitchhiker out of your life?

As you've seen in previous chapters, the answer (thank goodness!) is really quite simple: You don't need to *do* anything! Quite literally. Physically. You simply don't pick up the hitchhiker (you don't *do* smokes), and then you let the chips fall where they may. You decide to accept ---radically so— whatever happens as a result of simply *not doing anything*, of not picking up Mr. T. the hitchhiker!

How do you "not do" the hitchhiker?

It's very simple--- but let's go to another chapter --- drive back to the Easy Off Ramp -- to make it very clear.

[Note: The Back of the Bus discussion for this chapter will be found on page **252**.]

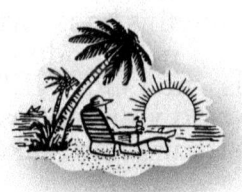

Chapter 13:
A Closer Look at the Hitchhiker

Any man who can drive safely while kissing a pretty girl is simply not giving the kiss the attention it deserves. --- Albert Einstein

Most of the time, for most of us, when we're driving down the road and see a hitchhiker, what do we do? We don't *do* anything! In fact, most of us pretend we don't even see the hitchhiker. We just drive on by. What do we have to *do* to not pick up a hitchhiker!

Duh. Nothing! Nothing at all.

This is the good news—and an often overlooked, over-complicated fact about quitting smoking. Again, for the hundredth time: Smoking is something that we *do*! Quitting smoking is not something that we *do*, it's something that we *cease* doing! (You've heard this before?)

Chapter 13: The Hitchhiker Up Close

What do you have to *do* to *not* pick up a hitchhiker? What do you have to *do* to not go bungee jumping? To not rob banks? To not sign up for mud wrestling? You don't have to *do* anything! Just relax. Be who you are. Don't *do* anything! Or even more simply, just keep doing whatever else you were doing! Just don't *do* the smokes --- don't do the bungee jumping, mud-wrestling. Don't *do,* just *be yourself,* (without *doing* smokes, without picking up the hitchhiker) and then let happen whatever happens.

Of course, if you've been picking up this hitchhiker (*doing* smokes) every day for years and years, we tend not to allow it to be this simple. We tend to pull over to the side of the road, lean across the seat, roll down the window and explain to the old hitchhiker, to our Mr. T. friend, why we aren't going to pick him up today. We maybe voice all of our complaints about his thieving behavior and his expensive ways and how enough is enough.

Mr. T., says, *okay, okay, sorry. I understand your complaints. So don't worry about picking me up. Don't worry about me. You don't have to pick me up right now. Not at all. I'll just wait. You go on, go ahead with your other business. I'll just wait right here. No problem. Sorry.* (Mr. T. will say anything at any time to stay in your good graces, because he's also a liar!)

So you drive away, but can't help yourself. You check him out in the rear view mirror. He's there grinning, nodding his head, watching you. He sees you check him out. He waves. Muscle memory kicks in. You wave back.

We know what happens from here. You go on about your business but that afternoon, or evening, or the next morning, whenever, you give in. You've been thinking about this mean, stupid, fickle hitchhiker constantly ever since you drove away. So, sooner or later, you drive back around to where he was standing, to where you left him.

Yep. He's still right there. You pull over and stop. He waves, grins, runs, opens your door, hops in. All is immediately forgiven, at least on his part. You two drive off again. He settles back in the passenger seat. It's your car, your gas, your time and your dime. He's back where he wants to be. He reaches in his shirt pocket, pulls out the pack. "Smoke?" he asks, grinning, offering you one. He already knows this is the only reason you came back to get him.

We've all been in this somewhat humbling, very annoying and secretly humiliating position. It seems as though we just can't quit the hitchhiker, Mr. T. Uggh.

So rather than trying to run away, let's turn around, take a closer look at him, see if we can understand how he operates. Surely he

Chapter 13: The Hitchhiker Up Close

must have some weakness that we can use to our own advantage, to finally get the upper hand, finally get rid of him.

To understand him better, let's ask—and hopefully answer—a few pertinent questions. Like where was this hitchhiker born? How did he grow up? What does he like to eat? What fuels him? What's his story? What's his hold? What is he getting from us? Answering these questions, even briefly, should help us gain the advantage, maybe loosen his grip, allow us to walk away.

Okay, where was he born? In one sense we could say he was born --- just a helpless baby --- when we had our first smoke. He didn't have a grip on us at that point. We could pick him up and put him down. We had to carry him around. And yet...

We didn't just make him up. We didn't just decide on our own to dry and cure the leaves of some strange wild plant, then roll them up, light them on fire and see if we might enjoy breathing in the smoke. We weren't that clever.

No. Mr. T. was prowling the earth long before we were born. He was waiting here for us. It wasn't just an accident that we ran into him. The documented history of how the tobacco companies purposefully, strategically market to kids is a whole other book. But Mr. T.

was here prowling the earth even before he went to work for the big tobacco companies.

For example, three days after he landed, Christopher Columbus wrote in his journal, *We found a man in a canoe going from Santa Maria to Fernandia. He had with him...some dried leaves which are in high value among them, for a quantity of it was brought to me at San Salvador.* The natives had been cultivating tobacco for centuries, perhaps millennia. Carvings of Mayan Emperors show some of them smoking!

Even if our parents and grandparents did not smoke, we were all nevertheless born into a well-developed, deeply ingrained smoking culture. From our earliest days we saw "grown-ups" -- including movie stars, many of whom we loved and admired --- smoking as if it were the most natural thing in the world. Since before we knew how to read, ubiquitous advertisements, both blatant and subtle had been encouraging us to smoke, assuring us that smoking is cool, sexy, adventurous. Although most smokers assume that their smoking --- their relationship with Mr. T --- is something very private, personal and unique, he is in fact an unrepentant philanderer, always looking for the next ride. He's been this way his whole life, before we ever met him! He tells us we're his one and only --- and when we're with him it feels like that, very personal and intimate. But he tells the same lies to everyone!

Here's more good news: when we leave him, refuse to pick him up, he doesn't really

Chapter 13: The Hitchhiker Up Close

care. (Actually, he never really did!) Another sucker (literally) will be along in a minute. We didn't invent Mr. T., the hitchhiker, so we don't have to uninvent him. We simply don't "do" him, don't play his silly games anymore!

So, the next questions --- how did he happen to grow up, to take up so much room, here in our own personal space? What does the guy eat, breathe? What fuels him? All of these questions can be answered in a single word: *attention*. Mr. T. lives, grows, walks, talks, dances, and continues to be a force in our lives all because of the *attention* we give him. Attention is a magical energy. **What we put our attention on, grows!**

Mr. T., the hitchhiker, is like a stalker of a Hollywood movie star, and *you* are the star! Such a stalker would of course love any positive attention he might get. He would love it if you the movie star said, "Come on in, let's hang out by the pool, my staff will bring us drinks." Mr. T. would not argue. He would grin, walk right in and hang around until the hearse pulls up.

More often, however, the stalker has a negative relationship with the star. "You again! I hate you! Get out of here. I'll call the cops! I'm getting a restraining order! I've hired body guards to beat you up and keep you away!"

Curiously, the stalker loves such scenes. When the star yells at him it confirms that the star knows he's alive, that he's part of her life! The stalker feels that he and the star *do* have a relationship, as negative as it may be. Here's the key: **the stalker (Mr. T.) doesn't care whether your attention is positive or negative!** He loves attention of *any* kind. Attention is his food, his very breath.

So how does this play out in our daily smoking lives? What does it look like?

Hanging out by the pool, having drinks is obvious. We just keep giving attention to Mr. T.—keep picking him up, from morning to night, inviting him in, making time, making room for him in everything we do. We start by giving him a little bit of attention first thing in the morning, and then give him bits of our attention all day long until right before we go to bed, where we give him one last "good night" attention. Some of us even wake in the night to give him just a bit more loving attention. This is normal operating procedure for many smokers.

On the other hand, we also take out restraining orders against him. We tell him we hate him. We tell ourselves we're not going to smoke—not going to pick up Mr. T. --- here or there or somewhere else. We talk about him to ourselves and to others. We tell our friends and family how horrible he is--- or they tell us. **We put a lot of negative attention on him, thinking that if we just give him enough negative attention he'll go away**. But he never does. He loves our attention. He *lives* on our attention, be it positive or negative.

Chapter 13: The Hitchhiker Up Close

Again, at this point we don't have to *do* anything about these observations. We're just studying Mr.T., seeing how he lives, how he ticks. One of the basic tactics in guerrilla warfare is to "know your enemy," scout him out, see where he goes, what his routines are. That's what we're doing here. And what we've just seen is that **Mr. T. lives on attention**. Another tactic in guerrilla warfare is to "cut the supply lines." We'll be doing that. But first, we needed to simply see where he gets his fuel.

We now know Mr. T's history --- he was here long before we arrived, just *pretending* to be a teenager. And we know where he's getting his fuel --- from the attention we give him every day. But we still have a few unanswered questions. What's his hold on *us*? Or let's make it personal. What's his hold on *me*. Why do I keep giving him my attention? Is it really just his stash of nicotine that I want, or am I getting something else from him? What stories does he keep telling me that I buy into, that I believe? I am exchanging my attention to get something from Mr. T. What is it? What am I getting?

To answer these questions, we'll need to drive this bus around the block again. Take a fresh look at Mr. T. and his fancy dressing gowns and dance steps. See why you keep going back to him. For that, of course, we'll need yet another chapter.

[Note: The Back of the Bus discussion for this chapter will be found on page **253**.]

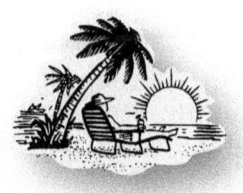

Chapter 14
Where attention goes, identity flows

"I feel when somebody has been playing cricket for a long time, he creates a separate identity for himself." ---- Sachin Tendulkar (One of the world's foremost cricket players)

Knowing what we do about Mr. T., why do we keep going back? What's his hold on us? Most smokers have at one time or another (or dozens of times) made a strong, clear, definite decision that they *are* going to quit, that they are *done* with smokes. They've had it with Mr. T. He's treated them so bad for so long they're completely fed up. They decide they're *finished* with Mr. T. once and for all.

And at the time it *feels* like a real decision. A true decision. And it's obviously the right decision. At the time it feels like "This is the *real me* making this decision" not to pick up Mr.T. ever again. *Ever!*

Chapter 14: Attention and Identity

And then an hour or a day or week later, it feels like there is a different "me" present. A "me" who really misses Mr. T., even though Mr. T. is fickle and mean and violently abusive. So we find ourselves driving around the neighborhood, coming closer and closer. Oh what the heck. There he is. We pull over. "Come on," we say, with a grudge. "Hop in."

So in that moment where was the *real me* --- the driver --- who a short time ago declared, *"That's enough. I'm done. I'm through with him. I'll never pick him up again!"* When we cave in and have a smoke, it feels like we're a completely different person --- at least in the moment --- from the *me*, "the decider" who a short time ago had firmly decided to quit. How does this switch in personalities happen? **How can we feel so completely different in such a short amount of time?**

Most of us blame this "switch" from *no* to *yes* to our own personal weakness, or to a lack of will power, or to being so hooked on these things that we can't stick with our simple decision to quit. After looking at it for many years, and working with many strong, highly competent and accomplished people who find themselves in this same boat, I would suggest our switch from *no* to *yes* is not the result of weakness or lack of will power or untamed addiction but rather due to **a subtle inner switch in identities**.

It's a very common, ordinary and observable switch that everybody experiences every day, whether they are smokers or not. When we recognize *how* this switch gets turned on and turned off, we will discover the key to freedom from Mr. T.

So, how does the "identity switch" get turned on and off?

Again, it comes down to one word: attention.

How Attention Works

Mr. T. obviously has a hold on our attention and won't let go. So let's set smokes and Mr. T. aside for a moment and just look at attention itself. (Yes, you can have a smoke, if you enjoy it, while we look at attention.)

Here's how attention works: Whatever we put our attention on brings up a story. The story brings up a feeling. The feeling brings up an action. And all of this can happen in less than a second. It looks like this:

Attention → Object → Story → Feeling → Action

To illustrate, and to keep this simple, and real, put your attention on something there in the room in which you are reading. It can be something mundane, like a plant, a lamp or a coffee cup, but the process will be more obvious

Chapter 14: Attention and Identity

if you put your attention on something like a photo, or a souvenir or a recent purchase. Let's say you put your attention on a photo of your dad.

When we put our **attention** on such a photo, on such an **object,** all the **stories** we have about our dad immediately come to the surface. If we've had a warm, loving and deep relationship with him then the **feelings** that accompany these stories are likewise warm and comforting. If our relationship was not so warm and comforting, then the stories and feelings are more conflicted, more troublesome. Either way, we may then decide to **act**, by calling him, or not calling him, or maybe e-mailing him, or if he's passed on then we might decide to call or e-mail a sibling. If the relationship was especially stressful we might act by deciding we don't need that damned photo sitting out all the time!

The simple point here is that when we look at the photo of our dad, it brings up stories and feelings and actions, even the action of avoidance, or non-action.

This same process happens a thousand times a day. We put our attention on something; that "something" brings up stories and feelings and actions. It can be something as mundane as a sink full of dirty dishes or as practical as our recent bank statement or as profound as a letter from an old lover. **Stories, feelings** and **actions** all start with where we put our **attention.**

Okay, let's look a little closer. Our personal stories are created by our thoughts and feelings. When the same stories--- thoughts and feelings--- rise up again and again, over and over, we start to *identify* with these stories. (Actually, most of us most of the time identify with all of our momentary thoughts and feelings, rather than with our more fundamental *being* in which all of our thoughts and feelings are arising. This tendency to identify with momentary thoughts and feelings, rather than with being itself, is a somewhat primitive, old-school, parochial approach to our inner and outer experiencing. Such limited identification --- with our momentary, passing thoughts and feelings --- is the root of all suffering. But this is a discussion for my next book, *How to Stop Suffering in Fifteen Easy Years*.)

We build up an identity around our stories. "I'm a Green Bay Packer fan," or "I'm not a morning person," or even "I'm a dad, or I'm a mom." And then, whenever our attention hits on something in that arena, this identity pops up. It looks like this:

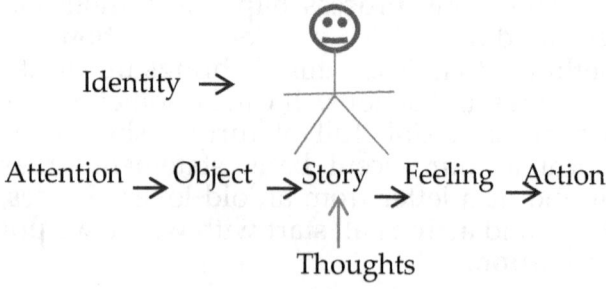

Chapter 14: Attention and Identity 119

We each have many, many of these identities, based on our stories, that rise up when occasion demands, e.g., when our attention is drawn there. We have our political identity, our spiritual identity, our "body" identity, our financial identity, sexual identity, family identity, tax-preparer identity and on and on. Our various identities remain mostly silent, invisible and dormant until "awakened" when our attention is caught on one thing or another.

Curiously these identities can disappear as quickly as they appear. A bunch of guys might be sitting around talking about last week's football game--- sharing and enjoying each other's *"football analyst"* identities--- when a pretty girl walks by flirting with her hips. The *football analyst identity* is immediately replaced (for most of the guys) by the *"lady appreciation identity."* And then if the boss walks into the room and the guys were supposed to have been working, both the *football analyst identity* and *the lady appreciation identity* are immediately replaced by the *"here I am working hard "* identity, or the *"here I am getting back to work"* identity.

Here's the principle: **Where attention goes, identity flows**.

Okay, back to smoking. Since you are this far into this book we can assume that you have a "smoker identity"--- yes, we can call it the hitchhiker, or Mr.T--- that "pops up" time and time again throughout the day, prompted by both internal and external cues. These cues--- and this identity—and the actions that come with it come into your daily experience through the avenue of your *attention*.

When you come to that place where you are ready to *stop doing* your smokes, you are basically saying that you are tired of playing with, responding to, the smoker identity. Although at the physical level you are of course walking away from the physical smokes, **what you are more fundamentally walking away from is the *smoker identity*!** In a word, you stop *doing* the smoker identity.

Easier said than done, you say. Remember all those times that you made the decision that you were *not doing* the smokes any more, and then, as we observed at the start of this chapter, sooner or later you were right back to it? Is it, as we have been taught, because the smoker identity is so strong, so ingrained, so difficult to walk away from? Or might the "switch" happen because of something simpler, and maybe sneakier?

As you might guess, I would suggest it is the "simpler, sneakier" explanation.

Mr. T.'s Secret Side:

The "switch" from *no* to *yes* (*no* I won't smoke, *yes* I will) happens because there's a little secret about the smoker identity—about Mr. T. the hitchhiker--- that he doesn't want you to know. It's a secret that I discovered only after closely watching him operate in myself and in my clients for several decades. I was very surprised when I finally saw it. Once I saw it, though, I thought—*duh*, why didn't I see it before? Here it is:

Your own Mr. T., your smoker identity, is two-faced. I mean *really* two-faced. Sneaky, sneaky, *sneaky* two-faced.

The face you know, of course, is the face that says, "*I want to have a smoke.*" Or "*I really need a smoke.*" We're all very familiar with this side of Mr. T. the hitchhiker's smoker identity.

We're all actually very familiar with Mr. T.'s other face, too, though we generally don't recognize it. Like I said, he's sneaky. He's a shape-shifter. So what is this other face, this sneaky side?

Before I tell you, let me warn you: This other face is going to be so familiar to you that at first you won't believe me. It'll be a little bit like finding out that your dear sainted Aunt Hazel has been embezzling from her Church's Poor People's Fund to finance her crack habit.

As a matter of fact, this "other face" of Mr. T. is so surprising, and yet so close at hand, that we best go to another chapter. You might want to sit down. You won't believe me.

[The Back of the Bus discussion for this chapter will be found on page **254**.]

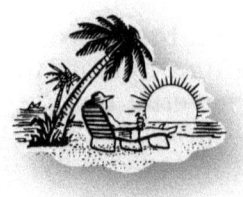

Chapter 15

Mr. T.'s Secret Face

"A man's true secrets are more secret to himself than they are to others." --- Paul Valery

I can hear you talking: Okay, let's have it. What is this sneaky other face of Mr. T., my hitchhiker- smoker-identity that I will find so hard to believe?

It's this: When you tell yourself, *"I really need to quit. These things are killing me! I swear, this time I'm really going to do it!"*--- **this** is Mr. T. speaking! This is his disguise! **The thoughts, the feelings, the actions around the idea, "I need to quit," are all expressions of the smoker identity!**

What? I hear you saying. *How can that be? That's my good side!* How can needing to quit possibly be the smoker identity? Are you saying that when I tell myself I need to quit that this is Mr. T. speaking? That can't be. Again, that's my

Chapter 15: Mr. T's Secret Face

good side. That *can't* be Mr. T., the smoker identity!

Didn't I mention that the smoker identity is really sneaky and two-faced?

Here's the deal: the *real* you, the natural you, the essence that you are, **your natural being doesn't need to quit because the real you has never been addicted**.

Staying with our metaphor--- the *driver-you* doesn't need to stop hitchhiking. It never was hitchhiking. The smoker identity is an added-on identity, not your natural identity. That's why it feels (at least occasionally) a bit *unnatural* to keep on smoking!

But let's back up, take this slow.

Again, when you say, as almost every smoker says at one time or another, *"That's it, I'm done, I'm finished, no more smokes for me,"* believe it or not, that's the hitchhiker talking, that's Mr. T. Or more precisely, that's one side of Mr. T.. He has two very distinct faces. One says *yes*, one says *no*.

Again, let's check out the old neighborhood where you first started smoking. Think back to when you first picked up Mr. T., when you first said *"Yes, I'll try it, see what it's like."* At the time Mr. T. seemed like an innocent, helpless little baby. It seemed you could easily pick him up or set him down. He certainly didn't have a life and death hold on you.

Okay, let's look more closely. At the same time that you said, *"Yes, I'll try it, see what it's like,"* there was another voice in the background that said, *"No, I shouldn't do this."* It may have been such a brief, quiet, unthreatening little voice--- maybe even a *giggling* little voice---that we either ignored it or pretended we didn't even hear it. Or maybe it was a loud strong "no" voice that we had been hearing for many years that we consciously decided to ignore. No blame either way. Let's remember, we were kids. Most of us did a lot of things when we were kids that we shouldn't do. But we were curious, full of life, exploring the world, looking for love and adventure. Welcome to earth.

The point here is that **both sides, both faces of Mr. T. have been here since the beginning.** And in the same way that *"I think I'll have a smoke"* has grown and gained power and strength through feeding it attention day after day, year after year, so too has the *"I need to quit"* been growing, gaining strength. You may have ignored the "I need to quit" side of Mr. T. for ten, twenty thirty years or more. But it's been there, in the background.

Most smokers get to the point where they say, Okay, I have been saying *yes* for long enough. It's time to start saying *no*. They assume that the way to quit is to take attention off of the *yes* and put it on to the *no*. We assume that if we just give enough attention to the *no* side, then the *yes* side will fade and go away. Again, Mr.T. is a stalker. He wants attention. He *lives* on attention. He doesn't really care whether it's positive attention (*yes* I'll have a smoke) or negative attention (*no*, I won't smoke.) Either way, our attention is on the smokes!

Let's look again at how attention works:

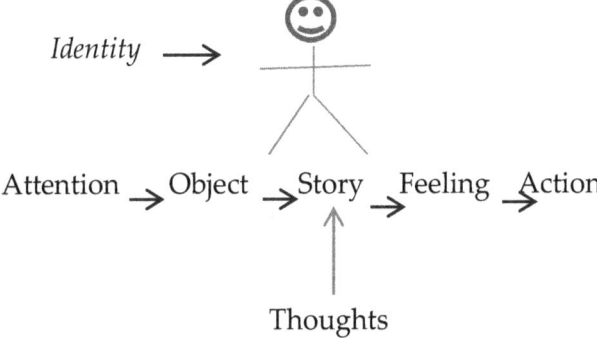

When the *object* we look at is smokes, it's going to bring up the smoker identity, and all the thoughts, feelings and actions associated with the smoker identity. Here's the key: **whether we are putting our attention on either smoking or not smoking (*yes* or *no*), in <u>both</u> cases we are still putting our attention on smoking**! And when we put our attention on smoking (or not smoking) we're going to bring up the hitchhiker, the smoker identity. When we think about *not* smoking--- put a lot of attention on *not* smoking--- we are pulling the switch, bringing up the smoker identity.

In my work with long-term smokers over the years it has become clear to me that our attraction to smokes is like a magnet, or gravitational pull. "Except with my coffee, I didn't have a smoke, and hardly even thought about having a smoke all day long," someone trying to quit will tell me, quite proud of their accomplishment. And then they will add, "Until after work. And then I just had one. And then not another one until after dinner, and then one right before bed. I'm down to just three or four a day. "

And yes, obviously, three or four smokes a day is much less damaging to the body than half a pack or a pack a day. And cutting back may indeed be part of the whole process of undoing the hitchhiker's hold on us.

And yet, as most people who "cut back" have experienced, *thoughts* about smoking and not smoking tend to continue quite consistently, and in many instances even increase. "Here I am *not smoking, not smoking, not smoking…*."

As we've discussed earlier, often the huge relief from having a smoke (*ahhh…*) comes from finally not having to *think* about the damned things, We don't have to think about whether we will smoke or not smoke! Having a smoke allows us to finally think about something *other* than smoking, at least for a moment.

Again, to be clear: when we think about *not* smoking, we're still giving attention to smoking, to Mr. T., the hitchhiker. The mistake most smokers make is assuming that when they are ready to quit they have to put a lot of attention, a lot of energy and emotion into *not smoking*. Knowing now that "no" is just the other side of Mr. T.'s *yes*, we can understand that when we are giving a lot of attention to "no" it's as if we are trying to recharge just the negative side of a battery.

No matter how much energy we are putting into *no*, we are subtly putting an equal amount into *yes*.

This explains how and why in one moment we can be very emphatic and determined, even passionate about "never smoking again," and then a short while later find ourselves lighting up as if we had never thought about quitting.

Obviously, quitting smoking is a big deal. When I quit smoking I wanted to put it on my tombstone: *"He Quit Smoking Before He Died!"* Yay. Quitting smoking felt like one of the major accomplishments of my adult life. For many people quitting smoking can be the difference between a long life or an early death. The difference between having money to pay the electric bill or not. The difference between a happy love life or no love life. Quitting smoking is, let's admit, a big deal.

Nevertheless, for all the reasons above, **our *strategy* for walking away from Mr. T., is to make it a non-event**. No big deal. We're driving down the road, see a hitchhiker, drive by, then see cows in the field and then change the radio station, then wonder if Aunt Harriet will serve her delicious peach pie. Saw a hitchhiker back there? No big deal.

With my clients the example I often give is, "I poured the cereal in the bowl, I quit smoking, and then I poured the milk." Two years from now, I tell them, when you look back and think about how you used to smoke, you can then make a big deal of quitting. As you're actually doing it, however, (actually, *not doing* the smokes) **as you're actually driving by Mr. T., make it a non-event**.

So okay, let's say we've come to the point where it's clear we don't want to pick up Mr. T., ever again, --- we don't want to *do* smoking any more, and we see why it's wise to make this whole process a non-event. What does that actually look like, moment to moment, and in the first days and weeks after quitting?

In the next chapter we'll look (again) at the absolutely easiest approach to "not picking up the hitchhiker" and how to make your experience easy and effortless. It's a two-step process, and in fact, you can be lazy (a slacker!) and not do the second step, because the second step will happen on its own.

With the exception of the chapter on quitting for health reasons, this whole approach has been easy so far, yes? Let's be brave, and just *keep* it easy.

[Note: The Back of the Bus discussion for this chapter will be found on page **255**.]

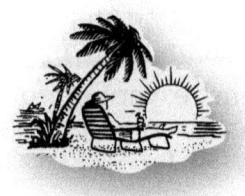

Chapter 16

Step One of the Two-Step *Not-Doing* Process

"Bad humor is an evasion of reality; Good humor is an acceptance of it."
                    ----Malcom Muggeridge

When we recognize we are tired of the smoking lifestyle, that we have come to the end of the smoking lifestyle, and want to take up the non-smoking lifestyle instead --- when we have come to the end of *doing* our smokes, and want to *not do* them any more --- what do we have to *do*?

Again, this is like asking what we have to *do* when we decide we're not going to continue our mud wrestling lifestyle any more, or we're not going to continue our bank robbing lifestyle. To abandon the mud wrestling or bank robbing lifestyles there's nothing we have to *do*!

Chapter 16: The <u>Not Doing</u> Process

In the exact same way, when we decide we're going to abandon the lifestyle of picking up hitchhikers alongside the road, what do we have to *do*?

Right. We don't have to *do* anything special at all. We just keep on driving, doing what we were already doing, being who we were already being. It's effortless. How much energy does it take to *not* pick up the damned hitchhiker? To *not* rob banks? *Not* mud wrestle?

Okay, granted, we know that all sorts of thoughts, feelings, sensations, worries and hopes are going to pop up when we don't pick up this particular hitchhiker. This is not just any hitchhiker. He's not a stranger. That's Mr. T. out there, our good-old buddy. (Well, at least our old buddy. He's not so good.)

We've been hanging with him for most of our lives. *Not* picking him up, just driving on by is going to trigger off a whole circus of thoughts, feelings, sensations, worries and expectations. It's like seeing our old abusive lover at the store.

So what do we *do* with all of these thoughts, feelings, sensations, urges, hopes, worries and fears that rise up when we cease picking up the hitchhiker? Again, seeing the hitchhiker is somewhat akin to seeing that a circus has come to town and set up its sideshow tents in our inner fields, our momentary experience. What do we do with this circus of sensations surrounding the hitchhiker?

Here's what we do:

1. Accept what's happening in the moment
2. Change the channel

Step one is we don't run away from the circus --- from *any* of our thoughts, feelings, sensations, worries, be they positive, negative or neutral. We don't run away from whatever is rising up in our experience in this moment. This is where our strategy of *radical acceptance* kicks in. We simply *accept* our experience in the moment, whatever it may be.

Let's be very clear. This step is very different than what is most often encouraged in most approaches to addiction. (And indeed, contrary to our cultural conditioning!) Most addiction treatment plans are designed around various smorgasbords of actions, of "doings" designed to avoid or diminish the often unpleasant thoughts, feelings and sensations that can rise up in the hours, days and weeks after stopping use of particular substances or behaviors.

The good news here is that we don't have to *do* anything about any of these unpleasant thoughts, feelings or sensations. **We simply let them be what they are. We don't encourage them, we don't reject them, we don't ignore them.** We don't exaggerate them, we don't diminish them. We simply let them be what they are.

In this way we simultaneously let ourselves simply *be* who we actually are in this moment. We don't fight ourselves or indulge ourselves. We cease to ignore ourselves. By accepting whatever is arising in our experience we allow ourselves to *be* who we already are in this moment. **We finally once again become friends with ourselves, by accepting ourselves, just as we are *right now*, without trying to change a thing.**

To repeat the quote from the start of this chapter, *"Bad humor is an evasion of reality; good humor is an acceptance of it."* The first reality we have to accept is the reality of our momentary experience, whatever it happens to be. We cease fighting it, cease fighting ourselves.

Easy, yes?

Easy, yet quite different from what we have been taught, and different from what most of us are doing most of the time, which is constantly trying to change and rearrange our inner and outer experiences. And especially relative to smoking, and quitting smoking, we have been offered a hundred different things we might *do* to change or resist or modify our experiences when we don't pick up the hitchhiker. But the *Easy Years* approach doesn't offer antidotes to our experiences. Rather, this approach is to simply accept (or *radically* accept) our momentary experience. We can *just be* with our various experiences. We don't magnify or diminish our momentary experience. We don't hold on or run away. **This approach is to *just be* who we naturally are in the moment**.

And yes, in some moments after not picking up the hitchhiker our thoughts and feelings might be quite tumultuous, even panicky. In other moments after not picking up the hitchhiker our thoughts and feelings will be quite hopeful, even ecstatic. Other moments will be quite mundane, as we pay the parking garage guy or fix our hair in the mirror. It makes no difference. We simply accept our experience in the moment. We don't fight ourselves. Both the panic and the ecstasy will pass.

This is a simple, yet liberating observation that is often overlooked: **both the panic and the ecstasy will pass**. Whatever we experience in the moments and hours and days after not picking up the hitchhiker --- all the thoughts, feelings, sensations, physical changes that arise in various moments in our being -- will also fall away. We don't have to *do* anything about any of them for them to fall away! Most of them will fall away within moments; others will fall away within minutes; a few rare sensations may hang on for as long as an hour. But life, like the river, keeps flowing. Most thoughts, feelings and sensations will come and go as easily, as smoothly as the passing wind.

Chapter 16: The <u>Not Doing</u> Process

What will not pass is our own familiar, ordinary being, our ordinary presence, and the constantly changing colors and tones and textures within and without. Step one in the moments after *not* picking up the hitchhiker is to simply accept ourselves just as we are---accept the river of feelings and sensations that rise and fall just as they are. We don't have to *do* anything about any of them. Just accept their coming and going, rising and falling. That's step one. Again, easy, yes?

Okay, I hear a few grumbles from the back of the bus. "No, it's not easy at all!"

Granted, if you've been smoking many years, and you are quitting cold turkey—not using nicotine patches or gum or lozenges, not using Chantix or Zyban --- your momentary bodily sensations may be quite animated for a few days. (By the way, research shows that *most* smokers who quit do so without using any of the stop smoking aids, contrary to what the television commercials might suggest. Most smokers quit cold turkey, e.g., *doing nothing*! Stop smoking aids may indeed be useful, especially if combined with a program where you can talk with others, but they are certainly not necessary, as millions of ex-smokers have proven over the years. We'll talk more about various stop smoking aids in Chapters 20, 21 and 22.)

For those who grumble that "doing nothing, just accepting" is *not* easy, let's take our bus on a short drive through the old neighborhood where we first started smoking. It's easy to remember that when we first took up the smoking lifestyle our bodies "talked" to us in ways that they hadn't talked before. For most of us, the new sensations of smoking were quite intense and animated, at times downright yucky, even nauseating, at other times somewhat pleasant and enticing.

"Hey, what are you doing up there?" our bodies asked, when we first sucked in the tobacco smoke. For most of us, our bodies resisted, rebelled. So we coughed, hacked, felt dizzy, nauseous.

Nevertheless, we grinned, laughed, encouraged these sensations. When we first started smoking, **we _accepted_, even welcomed the new sensations that came with this new lifestyle we were learning.** After a while, our bodies acquiesced. We no longer felt those early sensations. After a rough start, we had adopted a new lifestyle.

You can see where this discussion is heading. When we ditch the hitchhiker and take up this new non-smoking lifestyle, after years or decades of the smoking lifestyle, our bodies will probably indeed start to talk to us, offer up many new intense and animated sensations (a moment at a time). In various moments during our first days or weeks in this new lifestyle we may occasionally feel disoriented, or edgy, maybe even dizzy or weak

Chapter 16: The <u>Not Doing</u> Process

or hot or cold, tired or not able to sleep, or sleeping too much. What do we do about these new sensations?

We do nothing! We don't fight them. We don't exaggerate them or diminish them. We simply accept them, just as we accepted the new sensations when we first started smoking. We didn't have to *do* anything about the sensations—the thoughts, feelings, giggles, tears, worries, hopes --- that arose when we first started smoking.

And in the same way we don't have to *do* anything about the sensations --- thoughts, feelings, giggles, tears, worries, hopes ---- that arise when we take up this new *non-smoking* lifestyle.

Good news here: Your body is going to *love* this new lifestyle! Much more than the old lifestyle. Your body is going to quickly thank you. Rather than rebel, it will embrace this new lifestyle! Your body *loves* the non-smoking lifestyle. You can interpret any strange new sensations, feelings and bodily changes as your body coming back alive, dancing with delight!

Yes, of course our bodies and minds and emotions are going to act up when we cease picking up the hitchhiker. We can enjoy the acting up! In the same way we enjoyed (somewhat) the new sensations when we first started smoking. Enjoying the new sensations is the easiest way to deal with them. And if enjoying seems a bit much, then the second easiest way is to simply accept them, not fight them, not try to change or rearrange these new sensations.

We previously mentioned the stop-smoking guru Allen Carr, who wrote the best-selling book *Allen Carr's Easy Way to Stop Smoking*. Again, his basic advice for quitting?

1. Make the decision you will never smoke again.
2. Don't mope about it. Rejoice.

Another way of saying "Don't mope about it," is "Don't fight yourself or your sensations. Don't try to run away. Just accept —or better yet, *enjoy* --- what's rising up in the moment."

More good news here: You may not experience *any* strange or uncomfortable or unsettling new sensations, other than peace and contentment. It can be like having an overlong house guest who finally departs! Thank goodness! Whew! Finally. I get my life back!

"Hey Bear," one client complained, with a chuckle, over the phone. "Where are all these withdrawals I'm supposed to be going through? I don't feel anything, except relief! "

I've heard it time and time again. When we don't fight the sensations (or even label them as "withdrawals") and accept ourselves just as we are, enjoy ourselves as we are, life flows smoothly. Our new lifestyle becomes effortless.

Chapter 16: The <u>Not Doing</u> Process

So again, how do we take up this new "hitchhiker-less" lifestyle? It's easy. Step one is we don't *do* anything --- simply don't pick up the hitchhiker ---and then accept whatever happens, within and without. **Step one is to *accept ourselves as we are in this moment*.** What could be easier?

Step two, if we feel we really need to *do* something, is to simply change the channel. We move our attention onto any of a thousand different things. Not only move our attention, but allow ourselves to get engaged, get curious and involved with where we move our attention. To look deeper into this, let's move our attention to a new chapter…

[Note: The Back of the Bus discussion for this chapter will be found on page **260**.]

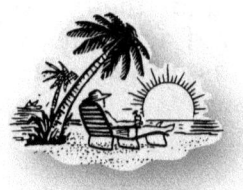

Chapter 17

Let's Pause, then Change the Channel

We can't plan life. All we can do is be available for it. --- Lauryn Hill

Before we change the channel, let's pause our bus trip here for a moment. We've covered a lot of territory. We're more than halfway through our trip, halfway through this book. It's time for a little refreshment.

As I said from the beginning, my intent here is to point out the absolutely easiest ways to quit smoking. I trust that many of you have been riding along, hopefully with a grin, or at least a relaxed interest, maybe nodding your head here and there in recognition as we point out things from our old neighborhoods, revisit old chums, remember how it was. *Ahh* yes.

However, having worked with many hundreds of smokers over the last several decades I also know that some of our fellow travelers here may be feeling a bit overwhelmed. What I myself consider to be "easy"--- simply accepting, not *doing* anything, giving ourselves more *ahh* moments, paying attention to attention and our various identities-- may seem quite heady and complicated to some. So what does this call for?

More good news of course.

The first good news is that **you don't have to know how to quit smoking before you quit smoking**! (You don't have to know how to *not do anything* before you *don't do* anything!)

Curiously, *most* smokers quit smoking without knowing how they do it! They come up with all sorts of explanations about how they did it *after* the fact, but as they are actually doing it --- actually walking away from the hitchhiker --- they *aren't doing anything*, they are *faking it*! Improvising. Making everything up as they go along. (In a later chapter we'll look at "improvising" as another way of talking about the quitting strategy in itself.)

The point here is, please don't worry about what you remember or don't remember about what you have read so far. Whatever easily sticks with you from these past chapters will be more than enough. You don't need to worry about what didn't stick, or what you've already forgotten. Again, **you don't have to know how to quit smoking before you quit smoking.** Just keep reading. It will happen.

Another piece of good news is that if you allow yourself to do the easy homework we suggested at the start of the book:

1. just be yourself, and enjoy smoking and/or enjoy not smoking;

2. just observe; and

3. give yourself more *ahh* moments

you will then find yourself easily, spontaneously doing what needs to be done to quit smoking, e.g, doing steps one and two. If you accept these easy assignments you will find yourself also accepting who you are in the moment and then spontaneously, effortlessly changing the channel and walking away from Mr. T., the hitchhiker. That early homework actually includes everything you need to know and do to walk away from the smokes. The catch here is that you actually have to *do* the homework! (*enjoy, observe, ahh.*)

"I was out walking," a client told me recently. "I really enjoy walking but I generally smoke all the time while I walk. I lit up my first cigarette and realized I didn't enjoy it so I put it out. I then walked for two more hours just looking around and enjoying the day. I didn't even think about a cigarette. At the end I was very surprised."

Chapter 17: Change the Channel

This dear lady has some deep mental and emotional challenges that her walking helps to ameliorate. For her to not smoke while walking for this amount of time was indeed a significant step for her. The point is that she made progress by simply tuning in to what she enjoyed and what she didn't enjoy in the moment. She allowed her joy to have a voice in her life. Joy works this way for everyone.

Further, when we are "just observing," not trying to change anything --- observing not only the outside world but also our own thoughts, feelings, sensations and actions --- we don't have any pressure to *do* anything. We will continue to do things—we can't help it. But our actions will be natural, easy, spontaneous, as easy as walking. We drop our agendas and live life as it happens.

And what's the feeling when the pressure is off? *Ahh...*

So just continue with the first three homework assignments --- enjoy yourself, and just observe, inside and out, and then in the process indulge yourself with more *ahh* moments. These simple homework assignments will lead to spontaneous dissolution of the smoking habit. Just watch.

Okay, then. Enough of this little refresher. Back on the bus... here we go....

How to Walk Away from the Hitchhiker:
Step Two: Change the Channel

Step one was to *accept whatever arises, inside and out*, after not picking up the hitchhiker. Step two is to change the channel.

Again, this second step happens anyway, happens naturally, effortlessly. This second step happens especially easily if we are neither pushing nor pulling our momentary experiences but rather simply *being* with them. The next natural location for attention will rise up on its own.

Still, when we *consciously* move our attention --- consciously change the channel -- we consciously, intentionally, take our attention *off* of Mr. T., the hitchhiker. In this way we drop the smoker identity, allowing any of our ten thousand other identities to function freely. How hard is it, and how long does it take when we are literally driving down the road and see a hitchhiker--- how long does it take to move our attention off that hitchhiker?

Right. Doesn't take any time at all, and it's easy.

In a previous chapter we looked closely at the mechanism of attention, and saw how, **where attention goes, identity flows**. By changing the channel, we change the identity. Mr. T. lives and breathes on the *attention* we give him. Again, whether we are consciously saying *yes* to smoking or consciously saying *no* to smoking --- either way, we are *still* consciously giving attention to smoking.

So what do we do? When Mr. T. pops up, we recognize him briefly, accept whatever feelings and sensations happen to rise up in that moment, and then let our attention move onto something else---anything else --- that is available in that moment.

Not only do we move our attention to something else, but we allow ourselves to get *curious* about that something else, or at least willingly engaged. Remember, **we are using the same gate to get out of the smoking lifestyle as we used to get in**. When we first started smoking we were at first curious, and then we willingly engaged.

What we put our attention on, other than Mr. T., doesn't have to be something special or grand or requiring a lot of energy. It can be something as everyday as watering a houseplant, or checking baseball scores or doing the dishes. In other words, we put our attention on our ordinary (hitchhiker-less) life. Although it doesn't have to be something special, it does have to be something immediately available in the moment when Mr. T. appears.

Again, when we see the hitchhiker alongside the road we don't have to make up something to do instead of picking him up. We just do what we are already doing. Since so many drivers smoke in the car, driving may be a good "case study" for how we find something else to do --- in the moment--- instead of smoking.

Let me repeat: **where we move our attention doesn't have to be grand or profound**. Let's say we're driving along and the urge to have a smoke rises up. We don't fight the urge, we just notice it, feel it, accept the feeling, and then change the channel, move our attention. Maybe an old rusty Oldsmobile is in the lane beside us. For a moment, we simply allow ourselves to get curious about the rust--- where it's showing up on the fenders, the hood, how it's progressing. We let ourselves imagine what it looked like when new, what it will look like sitting in the junk yard.

Sound silly? Yes, of course, but not as silly as lighting a match to some chemically treated dried weeds and sucking in and blowing out the smoke as we drive down the road. Obviously, we're not going to keep our attention on the Oldsmobile rust for very long. So then a semi-truck blows past. We allow ourselves to get curious about the wind patterns the semi creates for the other cars, or the out of state license plate or what it might be hauling.

The point is that *where* we move our attention doesn't have to be anything special or grand. It's the *process* of moving attention, and the willingness to be curious about the life around us that allows us to easily walk away from Mr. T.

Chapter 17: Change the Channel

Many, many times smokers have told me what they plan to *do* instead of smoking---crochet, or go for a run, or do woodworking, or clean out the closets. Absolutely nothing wrong with such plans, but how are you going to crochet or clean out the closet when you're driving down the road and have an urge to smoke?

Again, especially for people who are home alone, or home with kids much of the time, or who have regular smoking routines at work, deciding on a particular place or two to put attention in the days and weeks after not picking up the hitchhiker can be quite useful. I was recently talking with a mother of four who put together a thousand-piece jigsaw puzzle in the weeks after she quit. Another lady said she painted three bedrooms in the weeks after quitting. **Whether you move your attention to play or work doesn't matter. What matters is moving your attention**.

Still, too many smokers get caught on trying to decide *what exactly* they are going to do instead of smoking, assuming they need to come up with some particular activity that will replace smoking. This strategy is at the root of many failures.

"My plan was to go to the gym instead of smoking," one body-building client told me. "But I found that I really enjoyed a smoke after a good workout."

If we get too invested in *what* we're going to do instead of smoking --- where we're going to place our attention instead of smoking--- we lose sight of the basic and quite simple two step process behind quitting:

1. Accept whatever is arising in the moment
2. Change the channel, move attention.

When we recognize these two basic steps, we can engage them at any time and any place. We don't need any props, or special circumstances, or particular people (or the *absence* of particular people) to simply accept what's happing inside us. And then we can move our attention to something as easy and obvious as the weather patterns, or traffic patterns, or the different colors on the waxed apples at the supermarket.

As you can see, the first step--- accepting whatever is arising in the moment---is another way of saying *"Just be* who you already are." **Who you already are, is, at root, already free.**

If it seems as though I am suggesting that quitting smoking can in fact be easy, no big deal, something we do casually during the day, that's exactly right. For that, let's casually move to the next chapter.

[Note: The Back of the Bus discussion for this chapter will be found on page **262.**]

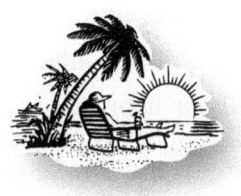

Chapter 18

The *No Big Deal* Strategy

It is our attitude at the beginning of a difficult task which, more than anything else, will affect its successful outcome. --- William James

As mentioned in a previous chapter, when I first quit smoking I wanted to engrave it on my tombstone.

BEAR QUIT SMOKING!
NOW HE CAN REST IN PEACE.

Quitting smoking felt like one of the major accomplishments of my entire adult life. And indeed, quitting smoking *is* a major accomplishment. It might even be a life or death issue. Of course it's a big deal. And yet...

During the season when you're actually doing it, when you're actually going through the gate, walking away from Mr. T., I encourage clients to make quitting a non-event.

How much of a non-event?

How much of a big deal do we make of not picking up a hitchhiker? That's how much of a big deal we should make of *not-doing* our smokes.

Here's why: **What we put our attention on, grows**.

Advertisers know this. That's why we get the same junk mail time and time again. Over a period of months we glance at it, throw it away. Glance at it, throw it away. Glance at it, throw away. Finally, about the fifth time we receive the mailer, we look at it and say to ourselves, "You know, I've actually been thinking about getting new siding for the house. Maybe I'll call."

What we forget is that the reason we've been thinking about new siding is because this advertiser has kept it coming to our attention! Of course we've been thinking about new siding!

The point here is, don't keep sending junk mailers to yourself about smoking, either for it or against it. Make it no big deal.

Chapter 18: The <u>No-Big Deal</u> Strategy

In trying to help people quit smoking, some noted health organizations recommend, "Tell everyone you know that you're quitting. " They do this because they assume that being held accountable by our friends and loved ones will help us quit. Or not wanting to disappoint them will motivate us. Or their words of encouragement will help. This may be true, on the surface.

"How are you doing with the quitting," friends ask.

"Doing just fine, thanks, until you asked."

At root, the smoking addiction --- and addictions in general --- are *addictions of attention.* When we tell everyone we know that we're quitting, then not only do we have to move our own attention off the hitchhiker, off smokes, we also have to move everybody else's attention. I'm confident that when our health agencies recognize the deeper roots of addiction, they will withdraw their encouragement to "tell everyone you know."

Many smokers worry that even if they themselves don't make a big deal about their quitting, that their smoking companions, or friends or family will certainly *not* allow them to make it a "non-event." Most smokers assume everybody else will see it as a big deal.

Not so.

Contrary to our own estimation of how gravely important our smoking is in our own lives, those around us, even our best smoker friends, regardless of how much they love us, aren't that invested, or even aware of our own personal smoking habits, or more precisely, our *non*-smoking habits. They may indeed be invested and aware of our smoking. But non-smoking? Curiously, they see our non-smoking as normal, no big deal, because, in fact *it is*!

My wife was not a smoker. When I quit smoking I didn't tell her what I was doing. Much to my surprise, it was *two weeks* before she noticed I wasn't smoking! To me, it was as if she hadn't noticed I didn't have a left leg! To her, seeing me not smoking was no big deal. She probably assumed I had just had one, or would have one soon. To not have a smoke in my hands did not seem unnatural. And in fact, it *is* quite natural not to smoke!

And even with our smoker friends and family, they won't necessarily notice. They too assume we just had one, or will have one. For us not to be smoking will not seem unusual to them.

For example, one of my clients, Maria, would get together with her three sisters four or five times a week. She was second to the oldest. They all smoked, and were all very close. When they got together they would drink coffee, smoke, and have nice long gab sessions about the people and events in their lives. They were

Chapter 18: The No-Big Deal Strategy 153

mature ladies, in their 40's and early 50', and had been doing this for a very long time.

When Maria quit, she told me she was not going to tell her sisters. "I'm going to see which one notices first," she said. Although Maria continued to participate in all of their regular gab sessions, it was not until *six weeks* later that one sister finally noticed, and even then she actually didn't notice. It happened when Maria was driving to the store with her sister. On the way her sister asked to borrow a smoke because she had run out.

"I don't have any," Maria said. "I quit."

"What? You quit?" the sister exclaimed, unbelieving. "When did you do that?"

"Six weeks ago."

Another client, a mother of three teenage girls, finally quit because they had been nagging her for years about her smoking.

"I think I'll start smoking again," she told me, half joking, a month or so after she quit. "When I first quit they told me how proud they were of me but after a few days it was as if I'd never smoked. They don't say anything. At least when I smoked I knew by their nagging that they loved me. "

Again, it's *normal* for us to not smoke. That's both good news and bad news. The bad news is that nobody ever congratulates us for being normal, or tells us how proud they are of us for being ordinary. The good news is that we don't have to carry around that old ball and chain! We can be normal again. What a relief!

As we discussed in the last chapters, the two-step process for quitting is first to *not do anything*, don't pick up the smokes, and then don't fight what rises up inside or outside. We first *accept* ourselves just as we are without the smokes. And then we change the channel. Move our attention onto anything else, and allow ourselves to become gently curious, mildly engaged with whatever else in our environment that our attention is attracted to.

Again, we're not going to get much applause for simply accepting ourselves and changing the channel. People may not even notice we're doing it unless we tell them. The fact that other people don't notice our quitting, or just notice briefly can be helpful. **Others not noticing can make the whole process much easier.**

This might be a good place to talk about our smoker friends who on the outside are encouraging and supportive but on the inside are quietly unbelieving and doubting.

Or maybe not so quietly. Sometimes our smoker friends can be obnoxious and challenging. *"You're quitting? Yea right. I'll believe it when I see it."* Or, *"Yea, how long will that last?"* We can expect such reactions from our smoker friends, and love them and accept

Chapter 18: The _No-Big Deal_ Strategy

them for their natural responses. They, too, are only human (and only channeling Mr T., the hitchhiker!)

And these types of responses are also why it's most often wise to make quitting a non-event. Our walking away from Mr. T. can actually feel threatening to some people.

Although we don't intend it in this way, our quitting may even feel like an insult, a "put down" for our smoking friends. No, of course that's not rational. But what's rational about smoking?

So again, let's keep it simple. Although we all know that quitting smoking, walking away from Mr. T. is in fact a very big deal, our _strategy_ while walking away is to make it a non-event, to make it very casual.

"I poured the cereal in the bowl. I quit smoking. And then I poured the milk."

That casual.

So. What do we do with our old smokes, once we walk away? Do we give them away? Flush them down the toilet? Put them in the trash? Or smoke them up to get them out of the house?

Glad you asked. For that, we'll need another chapter.

[Note: The Back of the Bus discussion for this chapter will be found on page **270**.]

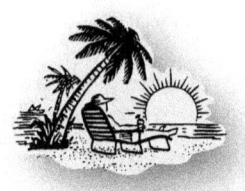

Chapter 19
What to Do With Your Smokes

The business schools reward difficult complex behavior more than simple behavior, but simple behavior is more effective. --- Warren Buffett

In California a number of years ago there was a run on cigarettes in thousands of stores. It was the day before a hefty new tobacco tax went into effect. Smokers wanted to stock up at the old prices.

At one of the big-box wholesale stores, a man (we'll call him *Sam*?) was seen pushing one of those flatbed carts toward the cashier. The cart was stacked with *boxes of cartons* of cigarettes.

"I'm just going to smoke these," Sam said. "And then I'm quitting."

Yes, of course, it seems silly when there are that many smokes in front of the guy. But how many of us have said the exact same thing, only with a smaller cart? *When I finish this pack, I'm done. These two packs. When I finish this carton, then I'll quit, be done.*

Or maybe we're not counting by packs or cartons, but rather by days or events. *When finals are over, then I'll quit. When my surgery is complete, then I'll quit. When the kids leave. When the kids come home. After football season. When things settle down at work. This summer. This winter. Before I'm forty, or sixty, or ninety, then I'll quit.*

In other words—*just five more packs, ten more packs, fifty packs, a hundred packs, then I'll quit.* When we look closely, we see that we aren't that much different from Sam at the warehouse pushing boxes of cartons. How many boxes of cartons have we already bought? If we piled them all on a flatbed cart, what would that look like?

Here's a secret: **"I'll quit when this pack is done" is Mr. T. talking.** The hitchhiker is very ready, even eager to quit later, be it thirty minutes from now or thirty days. It seems very reasonable, to him and to you, that you will indeed *quit later*.

Again, back to basics: the *only* time it's possible to not pick up the smokes --- to not do smokes --- is right now. The only time to *not do* anything --- to drive on by --- is right now. We can never drive on by *later*. In whatever moment we choose to *not do* cigarettes, that moment will be right now.

That's actually good news. It means we never have to wait, because it's always *right now*. We can settle in to *right now*. Be at ease with *right now*. Learn to enjoy *right now*.

So what do we do about the smokes we have in our possession right now?

Granted, most of us assume, because we've been told so, that it will be much easier to not pick up a smoke if we don't have any in the house, or in our pocket or purse. We've been told time and again by the medical experts that when we get ready to quit we should get rid of our smokes. Clean out all the ashtrays. Not have any in the house. Most every smoker assumes this is the way it "should be done."

But for most long term smokers, "not having any smokes" has been, for many, many years, viewed as an *emergency* circumstance. Almost a life and death catastrophe. Panic time. Totally unacceptable. Lights start blinking. Sirens blare:

"EMERGENCY! EMERGENCY! NO SMOKES! NO SMOKES! DROP WHAT YOU'RE DOING. GO GET SOME *NOW*!"

If this is how we've been viewing "no smokes" for so long, does it make sense to add this blaring psychological warning system to the "non-event" of not picking up the hitchhiker?

Here's a little secret: at root, **the presence or absence of smokes really has nothing to do with whether you smoke them**! Not having any smokes has nothing to do with *not doing* smokes!

This was driven home to me when my own mother finally quit smoking at age seventy-seven. (I used to tell her, "lay low, ma. Your son's a stop smoking coach.")

My mom had tried to quit for over fifty years. She said the way she finally did it (in addition to the great wisdom from her son, of course), was by leaving her smokes in the pantry. No smoking the last pack. No throwing them away. No hiding them out of reach. (She'd already tried all those strategies.) She left them in the pantry, right off the kitchen.

She ended up in a nursing home in her last years. When we were cleaning out her condo, years after she quit, her smokes were still in the pantry. When she passed on, (from complications, alas, of COPD) she hadn't had a smoke in seven years.

Having smokes around after quitting is not unusual. After I quit, my smokes were on our nightstand next to the bed for many months. When my farmer uncle quit, after fifty years of smoking, he still carried a pack in his front shirt pocket for many months. And obviously, if you're quitting when there are still other smokers in the family, smokes are always readily available.

As we've discussed in earlier chapters, the smoking addiction is not at root a *physical* addiction. If it were, the nicotine patches, gum and lozenges would work seventy, eighty, ninety percent of the time. Alas, success rates for these products are about the reverse of that.

Again, the smoking addiction is primarily an addiction of *attention*. Walking away from this addiction is primarily the art of managing attention. Not surprisingly, for many smokers, *not* having smokes keeps their attention locked on their smokes. Curiously, having smokes, as they have had for many years, allows many smokers to make *not doing* a non-event, and more easily, more gracefully move their attention elsewhere.

When clients tell me they are ready to quit smoking in the next day or two, I often ask how many smokes they have left. Most of them can tell me quite quickly, without looking. If they buy their cigarettes by the carton, they might tell me they're getting low, say just two packs left. If they buy two packs at a time, they might tell me they're down to just one pack. If they buy a pack at a time, they'll tell me they just bought it, or have half a pack left. **Every**

smoker knows the condition of his or her stash, and if he or she is about to run out!

Most smokers have an inner "security camera" monitoring their stash. It is a very rare smoker, or a very rare circumstance, when a smoker simply *forgets* that he or she has run out of smokes. When we're down to just a couple of smokes left in the pack, don't we get edgy and start looking around for the nearest convenience store, or supermarket?

As smokers we have spent years making sure we don't run out of smokes. Even smokers on the very lowest end of the economic ladder make sure they don't run out by buying loose tobacco and rolling papers. And when even these cost too much, they never forget they don't have any smokes. It's often the main thing on their mind, the "sign" that they've hit bottom, money-wise.

So, again, when we get ready to quit, do we want our inner security camera flashing red lights, and the sirens going off, "EMERGENCY! EMERGENCY! "? Haven't we just talked about making it a non-event?

Contrary to the official line, **for many smokers, keeping their smokes around can make it easier to quit!** No emergency lights go off.

Obviously, "keep your smokes at hand" is not a hard and fast rule, even as "get rid of your smokes" need not be a hard and fast rule.

Follow your joy. Some smokers refuse to accept the possibility that they could quit and still hold smokes. *"If I have 'em, I'll smoke 'em,"* they insist. So be it.

And yet, again, even when we get rid of all our smokes, finding another smoke is not a very high bar to get over—not much of a challenge. Stores selling cigarettes are everywhere. We can find them even at three in the morning. (And unlike alcohol, there's no curfew on selling cigarettes.) Or we could bum one from the neighbor who smokes. Or even a stranger. Yes, if we're in our pajamas and it's the middle of the night and snowing outside, we might not get dressed and go to the store for a pack of smokes. (Then again, we just might!)

By the way, **the most expensive thing you can do with your smokes is light them on fire**! I've heard it time and again: "These were too expensive. I don't want to waste them." The best way to *save* money is to not smoke them! First off, if you don't smoke them, you won't have to replace them. And if you don't smoke them, you'll be spending less money at the doctor's office, at the pharmacist, the cleaning supply store, the new clothes store.

Again, the most expensive thing you can do with your smokes is smoke them. So just let them be, right where they are. Go on about your life. Make it a non-event.

Chapter 19 What to Do with Your Smokes

So, I've put up a pretty good argument here for why it may be easier to "not do" smokes when you still have smokes to do. I need to repeat, though, that this is not a hard and fast rule. When I've suggested to some folks that they might not want to make a big deal of getting rid of their smokes, they immediately respond, "Impossible!"

I don't argue. Again, follow your joy, your peace. If it's easier for you to get rid of them by smoking them up or giving them to a friend or soaking them in the sink before throwing in the trash, do it that way. Even doing these somewhat drastic measures, I would encourage, if possible, making a non-event of it.

So the suggestion here: whether you let the smokes simply be, or get rid of them, in either case make it a non-event. No big deal. As William James was quoted at the start of the previous chapter, *It is our attitude at the beginning of a difficult task which, more than anything else, will affect its successful outcome."*

So it's no big deal whether you hold on to the smokes or get rid of them. No need to make a big deal of it, either way.

"Wait, wait," you might say. "We're getting very close to not doing smokes here. And I'm personally not that strong. Can't I use some help with this? What about those nicotine patches, nicotine gum or lozenges? How about

Zyban? Maybe Chantix? These are all proven to help smokers *not do* smokes. I've seen the commercials. Can't they help me?"

Sure they can, if you let them. Glad you asked. Let's go to another chapter, drive the bus around to the pharmacy, see what's on sale there.

[Note: The Back of the Bus discussion for this chapter will be found on page **271**.]

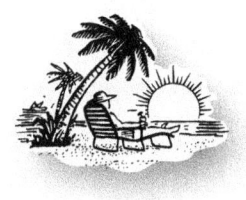

Chapter 20

Hook Me Up Doc--- I'm Ready to Quit

A doctor gave a man six months to live. The man couldn't pay his bill, so he gave him another six months. --- Henny Youngman

We started at the beginning of this book with the "absolutely easiest way" to quit (just be yourself and *not do* smokes.) We continued with next easiest way, and then the third easiest. We then did a quick detour to look at the hardest way to quit --quitting because of health reasons.

We've been taking this easy approach because not only is this approach more fun for me, your tour guide, and thus, I trust, for you, but also because the easiest approach is, not coincidentally, the most efficient. At some point, perhaps, we'll be forced to look at the *"fear, guilt and shame"* approach, which is another very hard and inefficient way to quit, even though fear, guilt and shame are quite popular and is the attitude most smokers (and their families and friends) try out first! Nevertheless, relative to our "easy years" plan, we're right on course.

So with that said, I trust you've noticed that we've covered a lot of ground before finally addressing the question of nicotine patches, gum, lozenges, and other "pharmaceutical aids" for quitting. This delay is not accidental.

Smoking is something we *do*, if I may remind you once again. Quitting smoking is not something we *do*. It's something we *cease* doing.

As we've discussed, our world culture is a *doing* culture, investing great faith in *doing, doing, doing* as a way to bring about personal and communal well-being, including personal and communal freedom. So when we're ready to *stop doing* something in our personal lives, we habitually look for something else we can *do* to help us stop *doing*!

The pharmaceutical companies are quick to jump in with suggestions.

It's not a conspiracy on their part. It really isn't. They, too, have bought deeply into the religion of *doing, doing, doing* to bring about well-being. They really do believe that *doing* their products will help you *stop doing* the smokes. In fact, they've spent millions of dollars *doing* research to prove their *doings* can help! And *doing* their products may indeed help. In the same way that day-laborers can help.

The Nicotine Patch, Gum and Lozenges.

Before we look at the more sophisticated (e.g., more expensive, prescription-based) pharmaceuticals designed to help smokers *stop doing* their smokes, let's first look at the common-man's over-the-counter solution: the nicotine patch, gum and lozenge. In the government-funded stop smoking program where I worked we gave out free nicotine patches, gum and lozenges as part of our six-session program. One of the obvious reasons we did this is because a deep literature exists documenting the decades-long research that confirms the efficacy of nicotine replacement products in helping smokers quit.

However, the research does not offer a 100% slam-dunk, no-brainer absolute certainty that these products help, and valid questions about the efficacy of these products ---perhaps even their harm --- have been raised by highly credentialed, well-established researchers. Nevertheless, on the whole, the accumulated research studying hundreds of thousands of smokers over many decades overwhelmingly suggests that yes, the nicotine patch, gum and/or lozenges do indeed help smokers quit. That's the obvious reason our program offered these products.

A not so obvious reason we did it is because we had discovered that advertising "free nicotine patches" was absolutely, without question the most effective way to attract new smokers into the program. Again, most of us are looking for something we can "do" to help us *stop doing* the smokes!

Curiously, many of the people who came into our program attracted by our "free patches" advertisement told me, in person, that the patches wouldn't work for them. Or the gum doesn't work, or the lozenges don't work. Many of these folks were hoping that maybe the other type would work --- if the patches hadn't worked, maybe the gum would. If the gum hadn't worked, maybe the lozenges would. If the lozenges didn't work, maybe... What can I *do* to help me *stop doing* the smokes?

Our program worked on a sliding fee scale so we tended to attract a high percentage of low income folks. As any smoker knows who has considered buying the patch, gum or lozenges as a substitute for buying all those expensive smokes, these nicotine replacement products are not necessarily a cheaper alternative. (If there's a conspiracy among the pharmaceutical companies --- and I'm not necessarily saying there is --- it's in the pricing of their products. Hmm...) That's why we attracted many people into our program who were looking for help in paying for the patches.

I offer this background by way of letting you know I'm not unfamiliar with the workings of the patch, gum, and lozenges. I've handed out tens of thousands of dollars worth of these products, maybe hundreds of thousands. In person, a week's worth at a time. And then on a daily basis I closely monitored the success, failures and in-between's of the people using these products.

What I told my clients as I handed out the patches, gum or lozenges is that these products work like day-laborers. I told them that if we have a *plan*, these guys can help us. If we don't have a plan, they wont.

For example, let's say we want to build a fence. We figure out how far the fence needs to go, in which direction, where it needs to turn, where the gate will be. And then we count how many posts we'll need, and stretchers, and we get our tools and materials ready. Then when the day laborers show up, we tell them the plan, show them the materials, show them what to do, how far to go. And then if the laborers aren't doing it the way we want it done, we can correct them, get them back on track.

But if we don't have a plan --- if we don't know if we want to build a fence or a chicken coop or a dog house --- then the day laborers will show up, just sit around, drink beer and smoke. Nothing will get done.

The point here is that when you use these products you're in charge, you're the boss, the foreman. The nicotine patches, gum, or lozenges can indeed help you quit smoking---help you *not do* smoking. That's your plan. But they can't *make* you *not do* smokes. No product, other than maybe a loaded .38 caliber hand gun, can force you to *not do* smokes.

So I told my clients if the nicotine products weren't helping them to *not do* smokes in the way they hoped they would, they were still in charge. I encouraged my clients to experiment, play around, try out different combinations until these "day laborers" actually helped them complete their plan, e.g., helped them *not do* smokes. .

Again, your plan is not about wearing nicotine patches or chewing nicotine gum. Your plan is to simply *stop doing* the smokes. Whether or not you are wearing patches, chewing gum, or sucking on lozenges, you still have to walk down the Easy Off Ramp on your own. These products are not going to walk through for you!

Again, no product can force you to *stop doing* the smokes. Even a .38 caliber revolver will be effective for a only a short while. (See my forthcoming, goofy, paranormal mystery novel, How to Stop Smoking in One Easy Second.)

More specifically, more technically, our plan is to take our attention off the hitchhiker. Our plan is to stop identifying with the hitchhiker, and take our life back. The subtly nice thing about the nicotine products --- other than giving our bodies the small amount of nicotine they have come to rely on --- is that these products give us a great *excuse* to drive on by the hitchhiker, Mr. T.   As we've discussed, at root it is the smoking *identity*, and not the nicotine itself, that keeps us coming back.

Here's why the nicotine products can help us stop doing smokes, but won't *make* us stop doing smokes: We're still going to see the hitchhiker standing there on the side of the road. **The smoking identity is still going to pop up regardless of how many patches we have stuck all over our body** and regardless of whether we have a mouth full of nicotine gum.

"Where attention goes, identity flows." So all the triggers are still going to be there, because our basic day-life patterns will continue as before. We will still wake up in the morning, (which is the first trigger for many smokers.) We may, or may not, continue with a morning cup of coffee, a big trigger for many smokers, but for sure we'll continue to commute to work, or continue to get the kids off to school. We'll continue to have morning breaks, official or unofficial. We'll continue to eat, and then finish eating—all very basic triggers for many smokers. At the end of the day we'll finish work --- another trigger, a time when many smokers smoke. We can't possibly change all of these basic routines in order to avoid triggers for smoking. Like it or not, we're going to see the hitchhiker wherever we go.

What many people are hoping will happen, or assume should happen, when they use the nicotine products is that these products will make the hitchhiker disappear. They don't. **The hitchhiker is a mental and emotional identity that does not dissolve with a patch.**

Nevertheless, I've heard time and again that the patches can help cut down the cravings. And the gum or lozenge is a good alternative when a craving arises. (Actually, the best way to use the gum or lozenge is pre-emptive---*before* a craving begins. When we grab a piece of gum or a lozenge in response to a craving we are setting ourselves up for long-term gum or lozenge habit. This is better than a smoking habit, but we don't want to be chained to any habit!)

Again, back to the plan: We're looking to *stop doing* smokes. We're looking for the Easy Off Ramp. How do we *stop doing* smokes? We don't need to *do* anything. We allow ourselves to *be* just as we are; we deeply accept ourselves just as we are.

The nicotine patch can give us a great excuse to "not do anything" when the hitchhiker pops up. It's like having another boyfriend or girlfriend with us when the old lover calls.

Intellectually, by wearing the patch we know we already have enough nicotine. So intellectually we know we don't need to *do* anything when we encounter smoking triggers, when Mr. T. shows up. That can be useful.

Chapter 20: Hook Me Up, Doc

And then the gum and lozenge offer us a momentary "alternative doing" to doing the smokes. In combination --- using both the patch and the gum (known in the biz as "combo therapy") we can have the best of both worlds.

Still, let's don't kid ourselves that we can *do* patches or gum or lozenges in order to *stop doing* the smokes. Whether we *do* these products or not, we still come to a point where we decide to simply *stop doing* the smokes. Whether we are with another lover or not, we still have to consciously decide we've had enough of Mr. T.

Because I worked for a program that offered these nicotine replacement products as part of the package, I've researched the literature deeply, and even talked with the researchers face to face. And then out in the field I've observed over many years how these products work, and don't work in smokers' daily circumstances. I know the politically correct "spiel" that goes with handing them out. If I hadn't been working for the program would I still have recommended using these products?

Not necessarily. Sometimes yes, sometimes no. If I hadn't been working for our program I wouldn't have been in a position where people were *expecting* to use these somewhat expensive products as part of their "not doing" process. In fact, prior to working for the program I did work for many years without recommending (or advising against) the use of these products.

These products tend to complicate the process. When I suggest there is *nothing to do* to quit smoking I know it may sound overly simplistic and naïve, but in fact it's the easiest, most direct and natural path available.

Although this direct approach is indeed simple, I'm *not* naïve. I've worked with thousands of smokers. I know that *doing* is something we have all been trained to expect, to focus on. So sometimes the patches, gum and lozenges help us to relax this expectation. In sales training there's an old maxim, *"First sell them what they want, then sell them what they need."* If someone wants a buggy whip, don't try to sell them a widget.

When people insist they want something *to do* to help them stop doing smokes, they can certainly *do* these products. What they need, however, is a simpler, deeper understanding of the freedom inherent in their own natural, ever-present *being*.

So what about Zyban and Chantix, the prescription drugs intended to help smokers quit? If we *do* those drugs, will they make us *stop doing* our smokes? Good question. Let's go to a new chapter.

[Note: The Back of the Bus discussion for this chapter will be found on page **274**.]

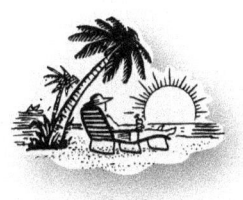

Chapter 21
Better living Through Chemistry

"A merry heart doeth good like medicine."
                    -- King Solomon

Okay, let's drive our bus down to the local drug store and see what goodies our local pharmacist might have to offer by way of help to overcome this crazy smoking addiction. After all, the drugstore is where most of us turn when life gets difficult. (Every year in just the U.S. alone, over 234 *billion* dollars is spent on prescription drugs.)

Again, we keep hoping for the magic bullet--- something we can *do* that will make us *stop doing* our smokes. In the weight-loss business they have the same hope: "We keep looking for something we can put in our mouths that will keep us from putting something in our mouths."

Obviously, if such a magic bullet existed, it would be worth many hundreds of millions, even billions of dollars. That's why the pharmaceutical companies keep experimenting, adding and subtracting, multiplying and dividing the whole rainbow of chemical molecules in search of the exact right combination that will help us *stop doing* what we no longer want to do. Although the pharmaceutical companies have not yet found the magic bullet, they nevertheless offer a number of "so-so" bullets that help some people, some of the time to stop doing what they no longer want to do, for a while. (My prejudices here may be showing through. The low success rate of most smoking cessation programs across the country, and across the world, with or without the use of pharmaceutical aids, should give us a clue that we've been barking up the wrong tree.)

So what are the so-so bullets?

Other than the nicotine replacement products, the two most popular, and widely used anti-smoking drugs are bupropion, (marketed as *Zyban*, for smokers, and *welbutrin* as an anti-depressant) and varenicline, (marketed as *Chantix* in the U.S. and *Champix* in Canada, Europe and other countries.) Before we discuss how each of these work, it might be wise to first look briefly at how they *don't* work, so that we know what it is we're looking at, and don't set ourselves up for later failure.

In studies submitted to the U.S. Food and Drug Administration for approval of these drugs for use in smoking cessation, it was found that after one year 10% of smokers who used a placebo drug were no longer smoking; 15% of those who had used bupropion were no longer smoking and 23% of those who had used verinicline were no longer smoking. (As of this writing --- late 2012--- even the 23% success rate for verinicline is being challenged by some outside researchers as higher than the data might support.)

Let's assume these figures for success are correct. These are the figures that the pharmaceutical companies use to advertise that their products will offer "fifty percent better chance of success," for quitting or "more than doubles your chance for success." Yes, that's true, and yet…

The figures show that more than eight out ten smokers did *not* permanently quit when using bupropion, or Zyban,. When using Chantix, more than seven out of ten did *not* quit. If we made automobiles, or toasters or light bulbs that had that high of a failure rate, we'd have an immediate recall! These bullets don't offer even close to a fifty percent success rate. And when we add in the potential harmful side-effects of these drugs, our faith in them naturally wanes.

Since my bias is already clear--that I don't believe these drugs address the roots of the addiction, in fairness I won't devote a lot of space discussing them. (That would be like asking a Ford salesman to present the case for a Chevy!)

Yes, these drugs can help, and have helped many smokers quit smoking, just as pinching off the heads of dandelions can help the lawn look better. And some of those dandelions with pinched off heads will even shrivel and die. Alas, such pinching is mostly temporary, and doesn't get to the root of the problem.

Buproprion- Wellbutrin--- Zyban

Okay, maybe my bias has led me to be a little unfair in my presentation of the data surrounding these drugs. The "success rate" figures that I shared are indeed accurate, but those figures were for success rates after a year. In the short term, the success rates are admittedly higher. Let's start with Buproprion, also known as Wellbutrin or Zyban.

Clinical studies found that in the short term (in the first seven weeks), smokers trying to quit who used Bupropion reported fewer and less intense cravings and withdrawal symptoms than those who were given a placebo. More specifically, "27% of subjects who received bupropion reported that an urge to smoke was

Chapter 21: Better Living through Chemistry

a problem, versus 56% of those who received a placebo. In the same study, 21% of the bupropion group reported mood swings, versus 32% of the placebo group." [2] Obviously, when we're ready to *stop doing* our smokes, fewer urges and mood swings, with less intense cravings can be a good thing!

Buproprion was originally developed and prescribed as an anti-depressant. It is still regularly prescribed for this purpose, especially in combination with other, somewhat more powerful anti-depressants. (On a side note, I've had many clients report that their insurance companies would not cover buproprion for use as an aid to quit smoking, so their physician would prescribe it as an anti-depressant. At some point, insurance companies may recognize that smoking is just as deleterious to one's health as is depression.)

Everybody (every *body*) reacts somewhat differently to different drugs, but in general the side effects of buproprion are mild. Nevertheless, at one point buproprion was withdrawn from the market because of the increased potential for seizures among users, especially among those who were using high

---

[2] (^ *a b* Tonnesen P, Tonstad S, Hjalmarson A, Lebargy F, Van Spiegel P I, Hider A, Sweet R, Townsend J (2003). "A multicentre, randomized, double-blind, placebo-controlled, 1-year study of bupropion SR for smoking cessation". *J Intern Med* **254** (2): 184–192. doi:10.1046/j.1365-2796.2003.01185.x. PMID 12859700.)

doses or were more prone to such events. In 2009 the FDA issued a health advisory, which warned that "the prescription of bupropion and varenicline for smoking cessation has been associated with reports about unusual behavior changes, agitation and hostility."

I had clients relate that they were able to quit smoking using Buproprion but the side effects were such that they had to quit using it, and then, alas, went back to smoking. Other clients have shared with me that they quit while using the drug but then, for completely different reasons, started up again. And then I have also worked with clients who were using bupropion during our six session program (one, to two to three months in duration) who successfully quit.

Let's be clear: there's no wrong way to quit smoking. Buproprion *can* help smokers quit. Again, like day-laborers can help build a fence or chicken coop. It's not a magic bullet, but if you have a plan --- an understanding of what you want to do (e.g., *stop doing* the smokes) this drug can help. It may be another tool to put into your tool kit.

I am actually quite tickled with the many millions of dollars spent in clinical trials to prove that the anti-depressant buproprion can aid smokers in quitting. My own take on it is that these pharmaceutical companies proved to all of us that **when people are a little happier they have a better chance for success**

in quitting than when they are a little depressed.

So let's give ourselves permission to enjoy the process. Whether or not we do it with the aid of "mama's little helper," a little pill, is not what's important. **What's important is that we give ourselves permission to start enjoying our daily lives more.** When we have granted ourselves permission for more little *ahh* moments, more *just being* moments, that which we *don't* enjoy will more easily fall away.

So much for the anti-depressant buproprion. What about the depressant, verinicline (Chantix or Champix)? This drug is designed to depress our enjoyment of smokes, so that we just don't feel like smoking any more. What's the deal with verinicline?

As depressing as it may be, we'll need another chapter for this discussion.

[Note: The Back of the Bus discussion for this chapter will be found on page **277.**]

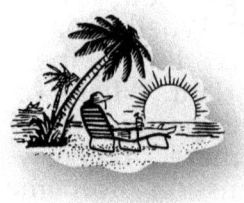

Chapter 22

Chantix : "It's Like Smoking a Carrot."

"I critique market-based medicine not because I haven't seen its heights but because I've seen its depths."---Paul Farmer

"*I*n all my 20 years in the business, I've never seen anything like it," one pharmaceutical salesman told another. He was talking about Chantix. He was grinning big and his eyes were shining.

I was at the National Conference on Tobacco or Health and just happened to overhear this private conversation between two well-dressed drug pushers --- oops, I mean pharmaceutical salesmen --- in the exhibitor's aisles. Obviously, I perked up my ears. Maybe they *had* found a magic bullet.

Come to find out, he was referring more to the commissions on his sales than effectiveness. In its first full year on the market, 2006-2007, worldwide sales of Chantix/Champix reached $883 million --- well over three-quarters of a billion dollars. (Good news for a commissioned salesman!)

Unfortunately, these early users were acting as unknowing "test subjects." Shortly after its introduction, reports started appearing about adverse side effects. Independent researchers started studying these reports from Chantix users and soon their findings were being published in various prestigious medical journals with warnings about possible dangers. This led the FDA to look closer and they soon ordered the manufacturer Pfizer to include additional label warnings.

In the U.S., media attention to the possible adverse side effects caused a steady decrease in sales of more than 33%, though sales in foreign countries did not suffer as much. European sales stayed strong and at one point in Japan, where one third of the adult male population are smokers, demand for Chantix far out-stripped the supply. Around the world everyone would love to find the magic bullet --- something we can *do*, to *not do* smokes.

How It Works

When first introduced by Pfizer, one of the world's dominant pharmaceutical companies, Chantix did indeed seem to be the magic bullet for smokers wanting to quit. In scientific terms, Chantix (verinicline) is known as a "nicotine receptor partial agonist," which for us ordinary folks means that it partially blocks the effects of nicotine on the brain. It is somewhat similar to someone grabbing a parking space right before we get to it. And then someone else grabbing the next parking space, and then the next one. Our joy in parking soon fades.

When using Chantix, nicotine can't find a place to park in the brain. The so-called "nicotine receptors," nicotine parking spaces, are all filled up. So on the one hand cravings are reduced --- the nicotine receptors are already filled because somebody (something) already has the parking space. And on the other hand the pleasure from nicotine is also reduced --- the pleasure derived from filling the parking spaces.

"It's like smoking a carrot," one of my long-term clients told me, sharing her experience of smoking a cigarette after taking Chantix for a month or two. Who wants to smoke a carrot? This old friend did indeed successfully quit smoking after using the drug (on the second go-around, several years after her first go-around.)

Other clients have reported similar successes. And still others report their expensive disappointment. And others, alas, report being totally freaked out by the side-effects.

At a fundamental level, when we start playing around with the brain's neuron receptors --- putting up roadblocks, mandating detours --- we've moved into an area of inexact science, to put it mildly. The brain is an amazingly plastic, wondrously mysterious living organism. But it doesn't include specialized rooms or dedicated highways specifically designed for enjoyment of nicotine. Scientists may find it convenient to label particular neuron switches and pathways "nicotine receptors" but that's just a convenient term describing a quite complex, multi-purpose biological function.

Calling these receptors "nicotine receptors" is like calling Wal-Mart the "tennis shoe store." Yes, we can indeed pick up a new pair of tennis shoes there. But a lot more is happening inside a Wal-Mart store than its function as a tennis-shoe distributor. So when we block the doors to Wal-Mart just so people won't be able to buy tennis shoes, we may indeed succeed in slowing the tennis-shoe purchasing, but we're risking simultaneously creating a hornet's nest of trouble both inside and outside the store.

Similarly, when we block the "nicotinic receptors" in the brain, we may actually succeed in reducing the pleasure gained from nicotine, but we're risking blocking the pleasure gained in many – or sometimes any --- other areas of our lives. And how is the brain going to respond to having some of its pathways blocked?

One of the most common side effects from taking Chantix is nausea --- e.g., the body wants to rid itself of this pill. Other reported but less common side-effects include headache, difficulty sleeping, abnormal dreams, flatulence and/or constipation. But these "normal" side effects are not what caught the FDA's attention.

In 2007, within a year or two after Chantix was made available as a prescription drug, the FDA started receiving reports that the additional effects of this drug were drowsiness and "erratic behavior." More seriously, however, were the reports of "suicidal ideation" (thoughts of suicide) and actual suicide attempts (and, alas, suicide successes).

In early 2008 the FDA issued an additional warning that, "it appears increasingly likely that there is an association between Chantix and serious neuropsychiatric symptoms." In the spring of 2008 Pfizer agreed and admitted, "some patients have reported changes in behavior, agitation, depressed mood, suicidal thoughts or actions." (Suicidal *actions*!)

In other words, **"we've been messing around with the brain's traffic patterns here and it appears that in response the brain sometimes starts to act a little wacky."**

With reports continuing to come in, in the summer of 2009 the FDA required Pfizer to place a "black box warning" on the packaging of Chantix. This is the most severe warning label issued, reserved for pharmaceuticals that can have very severe, even life-threating side-effects.

The warning --- which actually does appear inside a black box on the label --- is not without merit. In 2010 the medical journal PloS ONE performed a study that linked Chantix to a greater number of violent acts than any other prescription medicine on the market. That's worth repeating and put into black highlight, if not a black box: **Chantix is linked to a greater number of violent acts than any other prescription medicine on the market**. So much for the "magic bullet."

And then things got worse.

In the summer of 2011 the Canadian Medical Journal reported on double-blind research (the most rigorous kind) that indicated Chantix may cause heart problems, even for people who have never before experienced heart problems.

"[This research] would have raised a red flag," one government analyst said, "if the flag hadn't already been waving." The FDA was forced to issue yet another warning that verinicline, Chantix , may pose "a small, increased risk of certain cardiovascular adverse events in patients who have cardiovascular disease."

Pfizer responded that the reported research was too narrow, and didn't include enough subjects. So researchers went back, looked at a wide range of studies which included over 8,000 smokers. They kicked out all the smokers who had reported previous heart problems, and just looked at those who were normal. This left over 4,000 "heart-normal" smokers. Oh-oh. Chantix also seemed to cause heart problems among "normal" folks.

"I don't see how the FDA. can leave Chantix on the market," Dr. Curt D. Furberg, a Wake Forest medical professor and the senior author of the new report told the *New York Times*. Good question.

The basic reason that Chantix/Champix is still on the market is that the FDA considers smoking even more hazardous than all the potential side effects of this drug. So if it can actually help two or three out of ten to quit smoking, they suggest it's worth the risk.

What we need, I would suggest, is a much easier, much less dangerous way of quitting smoking, that would help nine out of ten, rather than two or three out of ten, to quit smoking . Maybe I should write a book...

Which takes us to another chapter....

[Note: The Back of the Bus discussion for this chapter will be found on page **281**.   ]

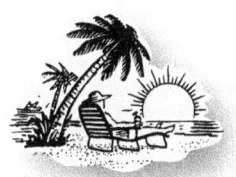

Chapter 23
Improv--- Just Make it Up

Life is a lot like jazz... it's best when you improvise. --- George Gershwin

*A*gain, there are no wrong ways to quit smoking.

In the U.S. a million smokers a year successfully quit smoking, and they do it a million different ways. (Actually, to be precise, each and every one of those million finally simply *stopped doing* smokes, though they arrived at the moment a million different ways.)

Obviously, there are easier ways and harder ways, elegant and inelegant ways. Going to jail, or to the hospital, or having both hands amputated are hard, inelegant ways of *not doing* smokes.

The point here is that if you are moved to experiment with Chantix or Zyban, I encourage you to do so. Nothing wrong with giving them a try. Obviously, I encourage you to enter the experiment knowing there are no magic bullets--- knowing that nothing will *make* you *stop doing* your smokes, though some aids can help. With such knowledge you can engage your experiment as an adventure, with a grin, and an open mind and hopefully a willingness to change course if need be.

What is necessary, and powerful is that we know where our experiments are heading: we simply want to *not do* smokes . We want to be hitchhiker-free. We're experimenting to discover how to most easily ditch the smoker lifestyle, ditch the smoker identity. Again, we are teaching ourselves how to *not do* the doing of smokes!

So how do we do that? How do we learn to *not do* the smokes? It may be helpful to remember that, from one perspective, on each of the Apollo space flights to the moon the modules were off course 97 percent of the time! The trips to the moon required tens of thousands of small "course corrections." One analyst calculated that for "every half hour the ship is in flight, it is on course for less than sixty seconds." Small moment-to-moment corrections were continuously necessary.

It's a bit like paddling a canoe. We paddle on both sides as a matter of "course corrections." If we just paddled on one side we would soon run aground, or be going in the exact opposite direction of what we originally intended. Small daily "course corrections" are a natural part of daily life. Doesn't it make sense that they are likewise a part of learning to *not do* smokes, to ditch the hitchhiker?

So how do we know which course correction to make? Here's a little secret: After we study and learn and read great books full of good advice, we then fake it, we just make it up, *improvise*. And if we fake, or improvise in one direction and discover we're a little off course, we don't give up on the experiment. We keep moving, and improvise in the other direction, until we reach our destination. Again, like paddling a canoe.

Let's go back to the million smokers a year who successfully quit smoking (who successfully "don't do" smokes.) Although they have many things in common as to "how" they eventually *stopped doing* smokes, when it came down to the daily life and actions that were *surrounding* their "not doing" each smoker had to personally *improvise* his or her way to freedom, or more precisely, improvise *in* freedom, since we *start* with *not doing*. So it makes sense that we could apply the same techniques they teach for improvisational theater to the process of *not-doing* smoking.

What? Improvisational theater?

Yes, let's drive this bus up to the local live theater and see if they might help.

I stumbled on to this idea when I came across the book ***Improv Wisdom***, *Don't Prepare Just Show Up*, by Patricia Ryan Madson, of the drama department at Stanford University. I was intrigued by the book for several reasons --- neither of which had to do with smoking.

First, for many years I was on the Board of Directors of our local theater company and books about tools and techniques for theater naturally catch my attention. But what really grabbed me was that somebody was purporting to *teach* how to do improvisational theater! I didn't know you could teach it. To me, that seemed a bit like trying to teach someone how to be spontaneous.

As I read the book, however, I realized yes, of course, there are principles and techniques for improvisational theater, just as there are principles and techniques for improvisational jazz or improvisational speeches or improvisational home repair. Some people are of course more naturally skilled than others at such improvising (think Robin Williams), but it is a skill that can be learned and improved upon.

As I delved deeper into the book it became obvious to me, undoubtedly because of my day-job as a stop smoking coach, that the principles outlined by Professor Madson for improvisational theater were the same principles every smokers used, consciously or not, to walk away from the smokes. Actually, Madson *intended* for the readers of her book to apply these principles in their day-lives. That was her primary purpose for writing it. I was just surprised at how neatly the principles applied to quitting smoking.

I highly recommend Professor Madson's book as a very life-positive addition to any library.[3] With her permission, here is a brief summary of eight principles she outlines in her book, particularly as they apply to walking away from the smokes.

1. Just say "*Yes!*" Perhaps *the* basic principle when doing improvisational theater with others is that when one character offers or puts forth an idea, a word or a twist to a scene, the other characters *never* reject or deny the idea. They always *say yes* to the idea, and then add to it. *"Ahh, I see you're a dentist." "Yes, I'm a dentist, and I only use a hammer and chisel." "Ahh, a hammer and chisel. That must make for speedy service!"*

Relative to smoking, *just say yes* to your idea, your urge to *not do* smokes, and then *just say yes* to whatever comes up. Say *yes* to yourself as you are in this moment, without the hitchhiker. *Say yes* to the *not-doing-smokes* experience. *"Just say yes"* is another way of describing the "radical acceptance" approach to our inner and outer experiencing.

2. Don't prepare How many times have we told ourselves that we aren't "prepared" to quit? The good news is that we don't need to

---

[3] *Improv Wisdom: Don't Prepare, Just Show Up*, by Patricia Ryan Madson, Bell Tower, 2005. Also available as an E-Book.

prepare! Preparing might even get in the way. When the time comes, we can fake it. We can just improvise

"Give up planning," Madson suggests. "*Clear* your mind instead of filling it….Substitute *attention* for preparation … if the notion of not being prepared is simply too much, try substituting the idea, 'Be prepared to let go,' or 'Be ready to go wherever things are going…Cultivate a flexible mind…"

From another perspective, we can easily assume that in our past years of getting to know the hitchhiker we have prepared quite well. When it comes to simply not picking up the hitchhiker--- not doing the smokes--- preparation and planning are secondary.

Again, here's Madson's suggestion: "Substitute Zen-like attention for planning. When you notice your mind is planning what you will do or say, *make a conscious shift of attention* to the present moment. Notice everything that is going on *now*. Attend to what others are saying or doing as if you would need to report it in detail to the CIA. Listen with both ears. Substitute attention to what *is* happening for attention to what *might* happen."

Using the concepts we've already approached in this book, we could paraphrase and say, "Substitute *just being* for planning." *Just be* with what is happening right now, don't try to change it; just accept it, inside and out. We don't need to fight it. We don't need to fight ourselves . We can just be with ourselves. We don't need to think too much about this. We can let go, feel what's happening, be present in the moment. We don't need to figure it out. We can *just be* with what is, here in the moment.

3. Just show up! As the writer L.M. Heroux put it, *"Stop talking. Start walking."* This is a very simple step, but very profound. "How often we avoid showing up for the things we need to do in life," Madson writes. She reminds us that Woody Allen suggested that "just showing up" is eighty percent of success. "Prerequisites such as motivation, desire, and warm fuzzy feelings aren't necessary," Madson says. "It is a con to imagine you must have these to get going…"

This is great news! Relative to smoking, "just showing up" for the game of *not doing*--- is eighty percent of success. It's akin to principle number one: "*Just say yes*." Just show up, just be right where you are, as you are.

4. Start Anywhere "All starting points are equally valid," Madson writes. She suggests we begin with what seems obvious in the moment, and then trust our mind, trust ourselves to edit and develop as we speak, as we perform. This seems obvious for improvisational theater, and it also seems obvious, and actually much easier for *not doing* our smokes. We just begin (we can *stop doing*) *anywhere*—and then trust ourselves to "perform." We can trust ourselves to spontaneously *do* what's necessary, what's "next" to continue in the process of *not-doing*. *This* is improv! We begin (to *not-do*) anywhere, and then make it up as we go along!

Perhaps a corollary to "begin anywhere," is "begin any time." Aren't we all looking for the exact right time, the exact right place to *stop doing* smokes? When we recognize that this *doing smoking* silliness is all theater, all a made-up game, then we are free to begin improvising anywhere and begin any time! There is no right time or wrong time. "Begin any time!"

5. Be Average Most people trying to learn improvisational theater are worried they won't be great, won't be genius, won't be funny. Madson helps them to relax by agreeing (*just say yes!*) to *not* being outstanding, great, perfect. It's okay to be average.

Same with not doing smokes. We don't need to be outstanding. We don't need to push ourselves, go for an A. We can settle for a C, and then not make a big deal of it. In this *not doing smokes* business, we need not be a star. We can be average, ordinary, and just not do it!

6. Pay Attention Madson suggests that life *is* attention. In teaching people improvisational theater she suggests people learn to control their attention, manage their attention (sound familiar?) so that they are able to place their attention on other people, on the surroundings, on what is happening *in the moment*! "Shift your attention from yourself to others," she suggests.

When *not doing* smokes this is the basic action! Relax, and then **shift attention.** Or as we put it earlier, *change channels*. Easy, yes?

7. Stay on course When folks are learning improv, they learn to stick with the particular scenes and/or characters that were first proposed. It's funnier that way, less confusing. "Keep an eye on where you are going," advises Madson, e.g., stick with the characters and the scenes you have built. "If you miss your target, adjust your aim." Get back to the characters and scenes.

So likewise, *not doing* smokes is like improv, only easier. When you miss the target, when you find yourself doing smokes --- simply get back to the play, get back on course! Again, we know where we're going here: we're *not doing* smokes. We're dropping that lifestyle, adopting a new lifestyle. When we find ourselves back in the old lifestyle, picking up the hitchhiker again, we can *start anywhere* and *begin again* this new lifestyle we yearn to engage. That's improv!

8. Enjoy the ride. People doing improv who aren't enjoying themselves aren't successful. Same with *not doing* smokes. Let's assume this is the last time in your life you'll be quitting smoking, saying goodbye to the hitchhiker.

Give yourself permission to enjoy the parting, enjoy the crazy adventure. "**Find joy in whatever you are doing,** " Madson writes, "**including ordinary tasks**,"

It is your *joy* in doing your ordinary tasks --- simply being who you already are in this moment --- that will cut the cravings, make the *not doing* of smokes easy. But also, "look for ways to play. Play is essential for human growth." *Not doing* **smokes *is* improvisational play!** Weren't we "improvising," just playing, when we first started smoking? Didn't we agree back in the first chapter that it would be easiest to get out of this maze using the same door we used to get in? Hmmm…

If you aren't too sure how to do this "improv" while not doing smokes, don't worry. Just make it up! However you do it will be perfect.

I mentioned at the beginning of this adventure that we would start with the absolutely easiest way to quit and then work our way up to more difficult approaches. We've been doing that. But "Improv"---just make it up -- is not that hard, is it?

So now we come to a few more difficult techniques- beginning with setting a quit date. When should we do that? Let's jump *now, right here, today* to our discussion of the quit date…

[NoteThe Back of the Bus discussion for this chapter will be found on page **284.**]

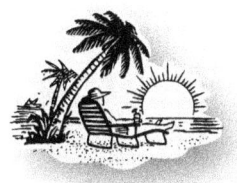

Chapter 24

To Set a Quit Date or Not — Is That the Question?

The best time to plant a tree was 20 years ago. The second best time is now. -- Chinese Proverb

Okay, should we or should we not set a quit date—or, to be more precise, a *"not do smokes* date"? To answer the question, at least partially, let's first drive this bus back to our old neighborhood where we first started *doing* smokes and ask a simple related question: Did we set a "start date" for smoking?

No. Not likely.

Invoking one of the principles from the last chapter ("start anywhere, anytime") didn't we just start smoking as a goof, somewhat spontaneously, as opportunity presented itself? Didn't we "just start anywhere?"

And didn't we agree early on in this adventure that it made sense for us to use the same door to get out of smoking that we used to get in? We didn't need a "start date" for entering the smoking lifestyle. Do we really need one to drop out of the lifestyle?

Most of the "authorities" would say yes, we do. The Centers for Disease Control, the American Cancer Society, the American Medical Association, the Quit Line all agree that setting a quit date is a good thing to do. They all encourage all their clients to set a quit date. And obviously, many tens of thousands of smokers — maybe hundreds of thousands of smokers --- have quit smoking (*stopped doing* smokes) by following this advice and setting a quit date.

"I'm a heavy-duty procrastinator," one of my young smoke-free clients claimed. "If I hadn't set a quit date, I never would have quit."

So be it. Absolutely nothing wrong with setting a quit date. Again, many, many smokers quit smoking by setting a quit date. Setting a quit date is standard operating procedure in the stop smoking biz. And yet...

Still other tens of thousands of smokers, maybe even hundreds or thousands —*millions*--- have set a quit date and then, alas, as the date approaches the stress increases and so does the number of smokes.

"I was getting way too stressed out about my quit date [coming up in three days]," a middle-aged woman client told me. "I knew I couldn't handle that much stress—or didn't want that much stress--- so I just quit right then."

She was able to use the stress about a quit date and turn it to her advantage. This is not generally the case. From my experience it appears that most smokers have set a quit date at one time or another and then for various reasons watched the date approach, get closer, closer, and then ---*arrghh* --- go on by. So they set another quit date --- watched it, too, come and go. And then maybe another…

Still other smokers never set a quit date because they fear failing. They somehow know, intuit, that they may be setting themselves up for failure. Who wants to do that?

"I hate setting quit dates," many smokers have confessed to me, based on their previous experiences. If quitting smoking --- *not doing* smokes --- is based in part on first doing something we hate, is this a healthy or workable approach? Or a slacker's approach?

And yet most smokers also assume that if they *don't* set a quit date, they will never quit smoking. That's what they've been taught. So they feel caught in a vicious circle. Welcome to the smoking lifestyle.

The reason professional health workers encourage setting a quit date is because they know that in smoking studies and randomized trials participants who set a quit date were more likely to quit than those who didn't. In the more enlightened of these studies participants were allowed to set their own quit date. In other studies, a quit date was set for them. In almost every scientific study the act of setting a quit date is assumed to be a necessary and important part of quitting. And again, participants in these studies who agreed to a quit date had a higher success rate for quitting.

So quit dates are actually necessary, yes?

This may be a good place to step back and again look at the larger picture. It will be useful to remind ourselves here of the generally low long-term success rates of almost *every* quit smoking program and the similarly low success rates found in various research studies. By "low" I mean that in 90 percent of these studies more than half fail to quit smoking, and more often it's two thirds or three fourths or more of the participants fail to quit smoking. Often it's a fifth (20%) or less of the people in these studies who actually *stop doing* their smokes for good.

Did eighty percent of the participants fail to set a quit date? Most of them did in fact set a quit date --- after all, setting a quit date was part of the process. They set a quit date, couldn't keep it, and then blamed themselves. (As did the researchers.)

So when researchers report that those who set a quit date are more successful than those who don't, they are covertly, or unknowingly simply referring to those who set a quit date and were able to follow the advice they were given, rather than the eight or nine who were unable to follow that advice, for one reason or another. **Is it in fact the fault of the smokers for not following the advice, or might it, just possibly, be faulty advice**?

In real life settings, outside of scientific studies and sponsored programs, do most smokers who quit actually set a quit date? After all, outside of these programs is indeed where *most* smokers quit! (Most smokers do not quit via a stop smoking program or a stop smoking study, though obviously I encourage such programs and studies. **Most smokers quit on their own, or often with the help of friends and family**, rather than in formal quit smoking programs.)

Curiously, very little research has been directed at discovering whether most smokers who quit in "real life" do so by setting a quit date. My own anecdotal evidence would suggest that most ordinary smokers who successfully quit do not set formal quit dates, though obviously many do (because that's what they were taught.)

This is also a good place to remember the Gallup survey that found that **most people change their behaviors not because of social pressure (quit dates?) or health concerns but rather because they are feeling good about themselves and want to feel still better.**

I would suggest that people who quit without a quit date do so simply because the opportunity to quit arises --- everything from getting sick, or somebody in their family getting sick, to finding a great new job, or having a grandbaby, or new lover, or losing an old one! As many opportunities as there are to start *doing* smokes, there are that many and ten times more for *not doing* smokes.

What I suggest to many of my clients who are fearful of setting a quit date is, rather than *setting* a quit date, *watch* for a quit date --- which I prefer to call a *"stop doing it"* date. I tell them that, obviously, if you have signed up for a stop smoking program (or if you've read this far in the book), there's something in you that is ready to stop doing smokes. The real work is to simply **get out of the way of your inner urge to *not do* smokes;** just let it happen, easily, naturally. Keep your eyes open—and your peace and joy at the forefront. It will become obvious--- that *this* is a good time, a good moment to simply not pick up the smokes. And from there, just *improvise!*

As we discussed in the last chapter, *any* time and *any* place can be workable. The skies don't need to open with trumpets blaring: THIS IS THE DAY! The trigger to *stop doing* the smokes, to drop the old lifestyle, can be something as simple as hearing a child's laughter or sharing a peaceable sunset with your spouse or simply being really, really tired of the struggle, tired of the freeloading hitchhiker's demands.

(The trigger can be something as simple as reading in a book that you don't need to wait for a *"quit date"* to stop doing your smokes! What a relief! What a non-event! How freeing!)

In my understanding the basic error in setting a quit date —a *stop doing it* date--- is that such a decision is based on the assumption that *at some later point you will be stronger, clearer, more adept, more courageous, more willing than you are right now.* This is simply not true. Said in reverse, you assume you are not now strong enough, clear enough, brave enough or willing enough to just *stop doing* these smokes. Again, this is simply not true.

Who we are right now, right here, is completely equipped to *do nothing*. We don't need to be braver, wiser, stronger than we are right now. **Who we are right now is perfectly capable of not picking up the hitchhiker, just as we were perfectly capable, as kids, of doing the opposite.**

Contrary to popular beliefs, it is in fact even easier to *not* pick up the hitchhiker --- to abandon the smoking lifestyle --- than it was to begin this lifestyle. All we have to do is....*nothing*!

And when do we *start* to do nothing? We can *start* to *do nothing* anywhere, anytime.

(You may remember that I have mentioned already that smoking is something that we *do*. Not smoking is not something we *do*. It's something we *cease* doing!)

And of course, if we are so inclined, we can also decide, "Next Tuesday at four I'm going to *start doing nothing*." Or, "On my birthday, I'm going to *start doing nothing*." Or, "when my stress level is down, I'm going to *start doing nothing*."

Let's don't make this more complicated than is necessary. Isn't it clear, when it comes to smoking, to not picking up the hitchhiker, we can start *doing nothing* anywhere, at any time?

Setting a quit date is another way of saying, "*I'm setting a date when I will <u>do-nothing</u>. It's my <u>do-nothing</u> date. On that date I won't do anything in regard to my smokes. I'll just be who I already am right here, right now. But on that date I'll <u>really</u> be who I already am right here right now.*"

Again, setting a "do-nothing" date for some date in the future is okay if that's what moves us. On that date we will "do nothing" about our smokes and allow ourselves --- accept ourselves --- to be just as we are. But let me point out that we are right now, right here already who we will be "up there." We are already fully equipped to simply *do nothing* about Mr. T., the hitchhiker. We are fully equipped to leave him begging beside the road, and go on about our ordinary lives without him.

Easy, yes?

So then what do we do, after we start *doing nothing*, after we drive on by Mr.T.? As the old Spanish proverb puts it, "It's wonderful to do nothing all day and then take a break afterwards." We can nourish the inner slacker. For that, though, we'll need another chapter...

[Note: The Back of the Bus discussion for this chapter will be found on page **285.**]

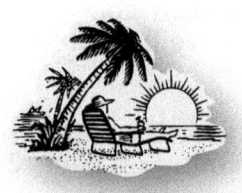

Chapter 25

Nourish the Inner Slacker

"Try to relax and enjoy the crisis."
                              --- Ashleigh Brilliant

Okay, so we've recognized that our freedom is closer than we ever dreamed possible. All we have to *do*, is *do nothing*! Just *be* who we already are, and let the hitchhiker fade into the background.

We see that just as we are we need not *do anything* about Mr. T., the hitchhiker. To experience our freedom we don't have to *be* anybody different than who we are right now.

So what should we *do* in the first days and weeks after *not doing* smokes, after dropping the hitchhiker? Other than be who we already are, of course, doing what we're already doing. After all, for most of us this hitchhiker has been riding along for a long time. Don't we have to *do* something special once he's gone?

As you'll discover, these first days when we are *not doing* smokes --- not picking up the hitchhiker ---- can feel a little strange. For many folks, they suddenly feel very peaceful, like we feel in our own home in the days after the departure of an overlong house guest. Whew! We have our lives back again!

On the other hand, the days after dropping the hitchhiker may feel quite wild, raucous, even exhilarating. Or they may just feel a little strange, scary, foreign. Especially for people who have smoked for 10, 20, 40 or even 50 years, *not doing smokes* can lead to feelings of emotional vulnerability, intellectual uncertainty and delicate physical sensitivity. So what should a person *do* in those first days and weeks when they are *not doing* smokes, when the hitchhiker is gone?

Again, in a word, *nothing*! Or next to nothing, as little as possible, at least interiorly. We could summarize this strategy as, "**Nourish the Inner Slacker.**" Here's how it works:

At its most basic level, when we are tempted to pick up a smoke, or a chew, just to make things easy on ourselves we can give ourselves permission for such an act. We don't fight ourselves. "I really want to do a smoke. Okay. I will." No fighting.

But then we allow ourselves to be a total slacker when it comes to actually following through, actually *doing* it. We just don't get around to it. We don't "do nothing" out of willpower or determination or necessity, but rather, just because we've given ourselves permission to be slackers. "Yea, I feel like picking up the hitchhiker but nah, it's too much work. I'm going to be a slacker."

And then we let ourselves get distracted by something else.

Next, we can be slackers when it comes to trying to judge how we're doing, and/or how we're going to do, with this whole "not doing smokes" business. We can allow ourselves to be lazy in our analysis. For the first time in a hundred years we don't need to figure the whole thing out. We just hang out with *what is*. We can be slackers.

And then when it comes to judging whether our family and friends are being helpful or not, with our smoking or anything else, we can be slackers again. We can forget to judge our friends and family, or just don't get around to it. (And when we do get around to judging people --- since this, too, is a long-habit for many of us --- we can give ourselves permission to quickly abandon the "judgment" work.) Same thing holds with co-workers and strangers on the street. During these days and weeks of *not doing* smokes --- of doing nothing about the hitchhiker --- we can be slackers when it comes to judging other people.

To make this easier, we can let our "people standards" drop real low for a while. Let's make it so that people can get away with murder, and careless driving and stupid clothes, as far as we're concerned. Let's let them be rude, or ugly. During the weeks, maybe months after abandoning the hitchhiker, when it comes to judging people, near and far, we're going to allow ourselves to be slackers. Being a slacker in the area of judging people just makes things easier.

We can also be slackers when it comes to all the "shoulds" in our lives. During these first days and weeks, let's slack away from the *shoulds*—I *should* mow the lawn, wash the dishes, paint the house. Doesn't mean we don't do these things. We can go ahead and mow the lawn if we feel like doing it, or paint the house or wash the dishes. We're doing these things, though, not because we *should*. We're doing these things only because we feel like it, because we are moved to such *doing*. In general, after walking away from the hitchhiker, we're going to be slackers when it comes to all the "*shoulds*" in our lives, at least for the first few weeks. We're going to cut ourselves some slack. **Let's grant ourselves a little easy-going freedom during these days. This is part of exploring a new lifestyle.**

In adopting this new lifestyle it seems wise and kind and empowering to cut ourselves a little slack—no, a *lot* of slack—in *every* area of our lives and especially in this one area of *not doing* the smokes, of not picking up the hitchhiker. After all, when it comes down to it, as we've discussed at length, all we need to *do* to not pick up the hitchhiker is *do nothing*. We've given ourselves permission to just be slackers when it comes to picking up tobacco, or even thinking about it. So it's fair, and helpful, to allow ourselves to be slackers in other areas of our lives, just for practice.

And once again, the essence of quitting smoking is not a matter of *doing* something, so much as *not* doing something. To *not* do something, we have to nourish the inner slacker. Granted, this is completely contrary to our modern way of life. Most of us are deeply addicted to *doing, doing, doing*. To suggest that we allow ourselves to be slackers is akin to allowing ourselves to be commies, or allowing ourselves to be rude, or self-centered. It's just not done. And yet…

Being a slacker is not being a commie, not being rude, not being self-centered. It's taking a moment to just feel what's true about our own lives as they appear right now. We're taking a moment to let life move on its own without our *pushing, pushing, pushing*. Just to see what happens. Just to allow the inner wires to get straightened out after so many years entangled with *doing, doing, doing*, and entangled with the hitchhiker.

When we allow ourselves to be slackers, a curious thing begins to happen. Yes, the laundry might be put off or the weeds might not get pulled right away. Yet we find other things happening, other things getting done that we hadn't considered. We find ourselves in the flow of life, where chores are accomplished without effort, without *pushing, pushing, pushing*. When we start nourishing the inner slacker, curiously, we find ourselves *more* efficient!

So what do we do after *not doing* our smokes, after ditching the hitchhiker? We allow ourselves to be lazy about judging, lazy about worrying, lazy about trying to get ahead, or fixing all the world's problems. In these days and weeks after the hitchhiker is gone, we give ourselves permission to smell the roses, watch the ball game, take in a movie, sleep late.

Although our strategy is to make this whole process a *non-event*, we know it *is* a big deal to have walked away from this abusive relationship. It is a life-changing, life-saving, life-positive deal. It's huge. So let's conserve our energy. Let's be brave. Nourish our inner slacker.

So where do we go from here?

We could come up with a grand finale, a stunning conclusion. Or just summarize the whole journey. Give one last trumpet blast of encouragement.

But we don't need to go anywhere. We can be just as we are, right here, right now. We don't need to try to make anything different. Let's just be slackers. Yes? Isn't that the absolutely easiest way to simply *not do* smoking?

Who you are is already enough. Just be yourself, and enjoy!

[Note: The Back of the Bus discussion for this chapter will be found on page **292**.]

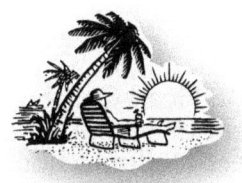

Conclusion
The Easy Exit Off Ramp

Sorry to say, happy to say, that's it, folks. The bus ride's over. We're back to the Easy Exit Off Ramp. This is where we got on. This is where we get off.

As you can see, we never actually left it. The Easy Exit Off Ramp has always been right here in front of our nose. It was so close most of us missed it because it was that easy to overlook. Come to find out, we don't have to *do* anything to not do smokes. We don't have to go anywhere than where we are right now. We don't have to be anybody different than we are right now. When it comes to fixing ourselves, we can just be slackers. Enjoy the day. Enjoy the fresh air. Enjoy the freedom.

Easy, yes?

Glad to have you aboard. Glad to have you exit. Feel free to contact me! I'd love to hear your stories, your questions and even your complaints. Mostly, of course, I'd love to hear that you quit!

>Bear Gebhardt, Head Coach
>Smokers Freedom School
>(www.smokersfreedomschool.com)

606 Hanna St. Fort Collins, CO. 80521

bear@smokersfreedomschool.com

In peace…. Bear

"I see the poem or novel ending with an open door."
                     --- Michael Ondaatje

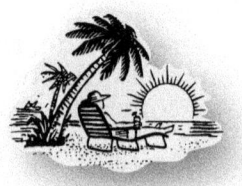

Back of the Bus

Dialogues

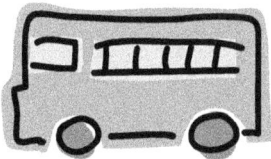

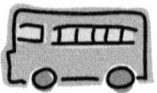

Back of the Bus: Chapter 1: How Do I Enjoy My Smokes?

Question: So okay, exactly how do I enjoy my smokes?

Answer: The same way you enjoy the rest of your life. By not getting caught up in your thoughts.

Q. Not getting caught up in my thoughts?

A. Right, not getting caught up in your thoughts. In fact, I encourage you to take it to the next step, and actually *enjoy* your thoughts. There's no other way. If we want to enjoy our lives, we have to enjoy our thoughts, not get caught up in them.

Q. Enjoy my thoughts?

A. Yep. Enjoy your thoughts.

Q. Thoughts about my smokes?

A. Yes, about your smokes, and anything else in your life that you want to enjoy. But since we're talking about smoking here, let's keep our focus on enjoying your thoughts about smoking.

Q. But I *don't* enjoy my thoughts about my smoking. I hate my smoking.

A. Yes. That's usually the case with long term smokers, and that's also why we started this book with this chapter, and your first homework. We're breaking some old patterns here.

Q. Okay. So how do I enjoy my thoughts about my smoking?

A. Ahh, glad you asked. It's actually very easy. Let me share a simple, four-part technique I learned decades ago from a French physician named Christian Almayrac. Dr. Almayrac was inspired to create this technique after meeting a renowned Indian sage named Babaji. When Dr. Almayrac asked Babaji what he should do with his life, Babaji laughed, threw back his arms and shouted *Be happy! Be happy! Be happy*!! So this became Dr. Almayrac's life's quest and after fifteen years he had invented and refined a technique that he called the *BeHappy* tool. I thought that sounded too corny, so in my first stop-smoking book I called it the Enlightenment Exercise, and in my second book I called it The French Technique, just because Dr. Alamayrac was from France. These days I'm calling it the Freedom Exercise. It starts on the next page:

The Freedom Exercise

1. The Law of Happiness: *Enjoying my happiness is the most important thing for me and for everybody else.*

2. The Link: *I enjoy my happiness when I enjoy the thoughts I'm thinking.*

3. The Question: *Whenever necessary, I ask, do I enjoy this thought, yes or no? If the answer is not an immediate and spontaneous yes, it's a no.*

4. The Action. *If the answer is yes (I enjoy this thought) I don't need to do anything. If the answer is no (I don't enjoy this thought) in order to return to happiness, I choose one of two options:*

  a. I drop the thought I don't enjoy to think and find or create a thought I enjoy more; or

  b. I choose to enjoy the thought which a moment before I didn't enjoy.

When you're enjoying your thoughts you're free. When you're not enjoying your thoughts, you're chained. It's that simple.

Q. So I'm supposed to enjoy my thoughts about smoking?

A. Yes. Exactly. If you don't enjoy your thoughts about smoking, you're not going to enjoy your smoking.

Q. But I *don't* enjoy my thoughts about smoking.

A. No, not yet. Very few people do.

Q. But if I enjoy my thoughts about smoking, won't I just smoke for the rest of my life?

A. No. Practicing your joy, not only about smoking but also in regards to everything else in your life, *always* leads to more harmony, more peace, more health, guaranteed. But let's look: Has *not* enjoying your thoughts about smoking led you to quit yet?

Q. Well, actually, a couple of times, yes.

A. Let me rephrase. Has *not* enjoying your thoughts about smoking led you to quit smoking permanently?

Q. Touche'.

A. I know this is a radical approach. We assume that if we just keep thinking scary, crummy thoughts about our smoking we'll quit. But from my experience, and your own experience, we can see it doesn't work that way. To enjoy your thoughts about smoking seems counter-intuitive, but I've seen it help people quit smoking time and time again. But if this exercise seems too hard, or too *woo-woo*, don't worry. Just tuck this little exercise into your back pocket and read on. Although this exercise is obviously very simple, and has helped thousands of people quit smoking, the book you're reading outlines an even simpler approach. So just pull out this exercise whenever it seems appropriate, but don't worry too much about it. Stick with the main program. You'll see. This is a no-pressure (and no-brainer) approach to quitting smoking, so if you really don't want to enjoy your smokes yet---really don't want to do your first homework—then don't do it! **Go ahead, be a crab about your smokes**. You're an adult, I assume, who gets to do whatever you want to do!

If you want to learn more about how to apply the Freedom Exercise to smoking, you can read my first book, *The Enlightened Smoker's Guide to Quitting*. But I'd suggest you read this book first, or instead. This book is a fresh approach, easier and more direct. Trust me. I've learned a lot in the last fifteen or twenty years about walking away from smoking.

Q. Trust you?

A. Or not. Follow your joy. And read on…

Q. This is already a very radical approach.

A. Yep. And the good news is, this approach works.

Q. I have to trust you that it works, right?

A. (Laughs.) Or not. Either way, my own happiness stays the same. But enough chatter. Let's get back to the party. It's only just begun. Let's read on. We're only up to chapter two.

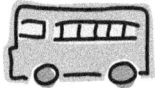

Back of the Bus Chapter 2: Every Smoker Uses the Same Exit?

Q. Did you just claim that every smoker uses the same exit to quit?

A. Yep.

Q. That's impossible.

A. Have you quit yet?

Q. No but...

A. Have you read the rest of the book yet?

Q. No but...

A. So relax, friend. Just keep reading. The single exit--- The Easy Off Ramp --- is much easier and more obvious than we tend to make it. And closer than the nose on your face. Trust me, all smokers use the same exit to get out of Smoke City.

Q. That's not what I hear, but okay...

A. Okay. Keep reading. You'll see.

Q. I'm a doubting Thomas.

A. I love doubting Thomas'. On we go, Thomas!

Back of the Bus Chapter 3
Are You Ever Going to Get to the Point of How to Quit?

Q. Get on with it, would you ? Aren't you ever going to get to the point of how to quit?

A. Yes. Sorry. But first, some more homework. Read on. (Oh, and by the way, just reading this book *is* how to quit!)

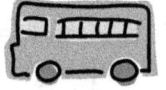

Back of the Bus Chapter 4: My Homework Is to Just *Observe*?

Q. I'm not too sure about this second homework assignment. My homework is to just look, observe?

A. Yep. That's it. Just look, observe.

Q. Observe the *ahh* moment?

A. Yes. that was the first thing we pointed out, from here at the top of the bus. But just observing our own patterns--- looking at what's really going on in our smoking lives--- is what this book is helping us to do. Simply by *seeing* what's really going on, we easily, spontaneously, effortlessly do what we need to do to walk away from the smokes.

Q. Again, I'm going to have to trust you on this, right?

A. Right. But you trust me by just looking, observing, see if it happens, see if it's true.

Q. I guess I can do that. One of the things I observe right off is that I don't have very many of those "*ahh*" moments when I smoke. I do have some, as you pointed out, but not very often. Most of the time it's just one smoke after another, out of habit.

A. That's a great observation in itself. *Ahh...*

Q. Very funny.

A. Sorry. But don't worry. You're not unusual in this lack of *ahh* moments. The reason many smokers smoke so much is because they aren't allowing themselves to get what they want to get out of smoking. They're habitually too busy *doing* something else. So they smoke one after the other.

Q. That's probably me. How I smoke.

A. It's most smokers. So be it. Don't try to *do* anything about this pattern. Just observe it. See it. The observation itself is very powerful.

Q. I guess I'll trust you in this.

A. Thanks. Hey *look,* on we go!

Q. Again, very funny.

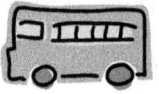

Back of the Bus Chapter 5:
Isn't This All Just a Bunch of Theory?

Q. Seems like you're putting out a whole lot of theory here and not a lot of practical stuff I can use for quitting smoking.

A. Actually, we haven't come to any theory yet. We're simply making observations. We've observed the *ahh* moment. We've observed that smoking is something we are *doing*. We've observed that quitting smoking isn't something we *do*, it's something we *cease* doing. We observed the transition from simply *being* as kids to *doing* as adults. These are things we can observe in our tangible everyday life, yes?

Q. Okay yes.

A. These simple observations, you will discover, help make quitting smoking much easier. Hang in there. One more chapter, and you're there.

Q. Just trust you, right?

A. Actually, no. I encourage you to test for yourself what I've observed in my own life and in the lives of others. See if these observations hold true in your own experience. I ask you to trust your own observations, your own looking, your own experiencing. That's the solid ground—no theory attached. Trust me.

Q. Very funny.

Back of the Bus: Chapter 6: *Just Be?* Are You Kidding?

Q. That's it? *Just be*? All of this has led up to *just be*?

A. Easy, yes?

Q. Actually, to be candid, I'm a bit disappointed. I can assure you, *just being* isn't going to stop me from smoking. It's not that simple. If it was that simple, I would have stopped smoking years ago.

A. Oh, for years during your daily affairs have you been taking the emphasis off of your *doing* and putting your emphasis on *just being*?

Q. No, of course not. But sorry, your suggestion here strikes me as overly simplistic, and somewhat silly. Again, I'm a bit disappointed.

A. Okay. Perfect. Thankfully, my job is not to try to change any of your responses. You feel disappointed, a bit irritated--- maybe I've been wasting your time--- and you're skeptical about this approach, yes?

Q. Yes. Sorry, but that's how I feel.

A. Perfect. And you say you're sorry because you don't want to hurt my feelings. That's nice. Thank you. I appreciate your honesty and candor. So, let me suggest, for just a brief moment, can you simply *just be* with these feelings of irritation, disappointment and skepticism?

Q. Just be with them?

A. Yes. Just be with them. You don't need to attempt to change your feelings, these honest responses. Or defend them, or even analyze them. These are your honest responses. So be it. This is who you are in this moment. I honor that. Can you *just be* with who you are in this moment?

Q. You mean *just be* pissed off?

A. (Laughs.) Yes. Just be pissed off. Can you cease fighting yourself, or me, for one moment, and just be with these feelings that have risen up in you? You don't need to exaggerate them or minimize them or explain them. Just be with them, as they present themselves, as they move through you. Can you *just be* with them for a moment?

Q (Pauses.) I suppose so. Yes.

A. (Also pauses.) So what happens when you do that?

Q. The feelings are not as intense. It's like they start to go away.

A,. Ahh… How does that feel?

Q. It feels okay. It feels good, actually.

A. Welcome to just being.

Q. Okay. I see something here that I didn't see before. But I still don't see how this will help me quit smoking.

A. That's okay. *Just be* with your not seeing, *just be* with your doubt. And read on. You'll see.

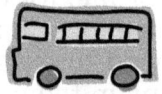

Back of the Bus Chapter 7: Radical Acceptance in Everyday Life?

Q. Okay. I'm starting to see what you mean by *just being*. Your idea of radical acceptance helps to make things more clear. But surely you aren't suggesting that everybody should just accept everything just the way it is. Nothing would ever get done. If everybody just accepted everything the way it is no improvements would ever get made. We'd all still be riding horses and buggies. Women wouldn't have the vote!

A. I'm not asking you to take my word for any of this. I'm asking you to just test it out--- test out what radical acceptance, just being *feels* like in your own life. See what happens in your own daily experience of the world when you stop fighting yourself. In my own experience when I stop fighting myself, when I allow myself to *just be* who I already am in any particular moment, I always discover more energy, more clarity and a quicker willingness to engage with various projects and with other people. And, in all humility, I have noticed that when I accept myself for who I am I seem to have more skill in doing what I do.

Q. I don't get it.

A. A wider intelligence, and greater energy begin to function when we stop putting on the brakes, when we stop trying to change ourselves and others. In other words, when we begin to accept ourselves for who we are, accept the good, the bad, the ugly, then the beautiful, natural intelligence has room to function.

Q. So I accept myself as a smoker?

A. That's your description of yourself in this moment, yes?

Q. Yes. Not only a description, it's a fact.

A. How long have you been fighting this description, this fact?

Q. A long time.

A. As the kids say these days, how has that worked for you so far?

Q. (Laughs) Okay. Granted. Not that well. I'm still smoking.

A. Smoking itself is the outer expression of an ongoing inner fight--- *I want to, I don't want to. I can quit, I can't quit. I'm fearful what it's doing to me. It might not be that bad. I don't care what other people think about my smoking. Oh shoot. What will other people think?* Yay, nay, all day long, yes? Does this inner argument sound familiar?

Q. (Laughs again.) Yea, yea. You nailed it.

A. Curiously, the easiest way out of this fight is to simply cease fighting. Be at peace with both sides. Napoleon said, "The only way the wars will end is when the soldiers refuse to fight." We assume our smoking wars will end if we just give the general on the quitting side a lot more ammo.

Q. Yes. That's what I've been trying to do.

A. Here's a little known secret: When we give ammo to one side, the other side steals it. We have traitors on both sides who hand the ammo over to the enemy. So what we do, we simply cease giving ammo--- giving energy--- to either side. It's actually a great relief.

Q. What do you mean? How do we cease giving ammo to either side?

A. By *just being* with whatever rises up. Deeply accepting whatever rises up in us in the moment. We accept all of our thoughts, feelings, sensations, actions, not only about smoking, but about everything. This means we cease trying to suppress our thoughts, feelings, emotions, but also don't give them any more energy than they already have. We don't try to change or rearrange our experience in the moment. This is *just being*. Deep acceptance.

Q. If we didn't do any of that, wouldn't we just become automatons?

A. My experience is, that when cease fighting ourselves we *cease* being automatons. We come more alive, more alert, more present with life as it is.

Q. Hmm....

A. Again, I'm not asking you to believe anything I'm saying here. I'm not asking you to take up another philosophy. I'm encouraging you to experiment with this--- allow yourself to be exactly who you are in this moment. For a moment, don't fight yourself. *Just be.* Accept what comes up and see what happens.

Q. It seems too easy.

A. (Laughs.) Yes. Actually that's been my biggest challenge in sharing this. It seems too easy. People assume, "If it was that easy I would have done it years ago."

Q. Hmm. That sounds familiar.

A. The challenge here is to learn again to be friends with ourselves, as we were when we were kids. As kids, we were happy to *just be*. Young children have a deep, profound acceptance of who they are in any given moment, until they are taught that who they are is not good enough, strong enough, big enough, fast enough, smart enough. It's time to become friends with ourselves again, like we were when we were kids. It's time to let the wars come to an end.

Q. Hmm. I like it. I'll try it.

A. There's no effort involved. It's effortless. Just be. Accept who you are.

Q. Yes. Thank you.

A. You're welcome. I like my work because I basically get to remind people of what they already know.

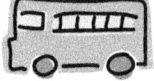

Back of the Bus: Chapter 8: Checking Your Homework

Q. Sorry to say it, but you sure repeat yourself a lot.

A. Yes, Intentionally so, thank you. Yes, intentionally so, thank you.

Q. Very funny.

A. Left brain learning is linear, logical. We add one thought, idea, onto another. Right brain learning is more circular, and often paradoxical. We come back around, look at the same things from a different perspective. We need both types of learning in this process. Smoking, as you may have noticed, is not exactly logical, or the result of linear thinking.

Q. Granted.

A. Bear with me. This simple approach to quitting smoking needs to cut through a lot of old programming. That's why repetition is necessary. A single sentence, a single insight may be enough to do the trick for you. I've seen this happen time and again. But you might have to hear this same insight, even this same sentence, time and again before the simple and beautiful reality behind the words, towards which the words are pointing, reveals itself.

Q. So just trust you, right?

A. (Laughs) You've heard that before?

Back of the Bus: Chapter 9: More *Ahh* Moments

Q. I've come back and reread this chapter because I realized I don't really have very many *ahh* moments. What you say makes sense, but my life is very stressful right now. After reading this chapter I realized I get most of my *ahh* moments, sometimes I think all of my *ahh* moments, from my smokes. Any suggestions?

A. Thank you. What you share here is actually a very profound insight. It shows that you are actually *observing* in your own life what is being pointed to. And you can guess what my first suggestion is going to be: for a moment, simply *accept* this feeling, this insight that you don't have very many *ahh* moments in your life outside of smoking.

Q. Accept that I don't have any *ahh* moments?

A. Isn't that what you just said? Isn't this what your experience is in this moment?

Q. Yes, but...

A. No but's. We're sticking with our real life experiences here. We're building on real life experience. Your experience, as you shared it, is that you have no *ahh*'s, or few *ahh*'s, outside of smoking. Yes?

Q. Yes.

A. So okay, just be with that for a moment. Don't fight it. Be brave enough to be who you are, right now.

Q. Without an *ahh*?

A. An *ahh* arises, as you will remember, when for just a moment we are content and brave enough to simply be who we are, doing what we are doing, even when it's something we shouldn't be doing.

Q. (laughs) Like smoking.

A. Like smoking.

Q. But I *enjoy* that *ahh* moment from the first puff of my smoke

A. Sometimes.

Q. Right. Sometimes. But it's my enjoyment that makes it an *ahh* moment. I'm getting a certain pleasure there. The recognition that I don't have many *ahh* moments outside of my smoking is not very enjoyable.

A. Granted. But let's freeze frame that thought for a moment --- that *not having many ahh moments outside of smoking is not very enjoyable.* What we tend to do is judge ourselves and try to fix it. *There must be something wrong with me if my only pleasure in life comes from smoking. What can I do to have more ahh moments?* When we judge ourselves and try to fix ourselves we are moving away from ourselves! It's very paradoxical.

Q. I think I see where you're going with this. But please, continue…

A. The original thought was, "*I don't have very many ahh moments outside of smoking.*" To *just be* with that, accept that, not fight it…

Q. *Ahh*….

A. (laughs) Exactly!

Q. Okay, yes. I'm starting to see.

A. I'll repeat: we experience *ahh* moments when we stop fighting ourselves, allow ourselves to just be where we are, doing what we're doing, feeling what we're feeling. As we just demonstrated here, we can do it anywhere, at any time, with anything, even with the insight *I don't have very many ahh moments*. We're *always* being exactly what we are and who we are in every moment. So any moment is an opportunity for an *ahh* moment. Every moment is an opportunity for an *ahh* moment. But we don't have to put such pressure on ourselves. We don't have to make every moment an *ahh* moment. Just whenever we remember to do so.

Q. Okay. So an *ahh* moment doesn't have to be something great and wonderful. It can be any moment.

A. Exactly. That's why we start with "baby *ahh*" moments.

Q. Okay, yes. So just sitting here talking with you can be an *ahh* moment.

A. Ahh...

Q. Yea, yea, yea. Very funny. But I see what you're getting at. It's not really the *ahh*. It's the accepting of who we are in any particular moment. Not fighting ourselves. Allowing ourselves to be who we are.

A. And again, *ahh*...

Q. Yes, okay. Now I get it. *Ahh*... Thank you.

A. *Ahh*, you're welcome.

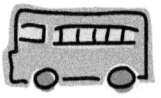

Back of the Bus Chapter 10: Quitting for Health Reasons

Q. Wait a minute, before you leave this topic, quitting for health reasons. I don't get it. If smoking didn't cause health problems, I'd smoke until I died. I wouldn't quit.

A. Hmm. Are you still smoking?

Q. Yes.

A. And do you know when are you going to die? Do you have a die date?

Q. (Laughs, nervously) Well, not exactly no.

A. So it could be tomorrow. Could be fifty years from now.

Q. Right.

A. So there's a possibility that you might *already* be smoking until you died?

Q. Okay. Touché. But still… Seems like health reasons are really the only reasons I want to quit. Well, and the money. And the social hassle. But primarily for health. If it wasn't for what smoking was doing to my health, I could deal with the other things.

A. Again, let's be clear: Quitting for health reasons is perfectly legitimate. Even if you quit for some other reason --- a new girlfriend, or new job, or it's just costing too much --- still, you would get all the same health benefits from quitting as if health reasons were your only reasons for quitting. Absolutely nothing wrong with quitting for health reasons.

Q. Okay, good. I just got the impression, from that last chapter, that you were poo-pooing health as a reason for quitting.

A. Health is obviously a very good reason for quitting. No argument. What I was pointing out is that although health is a good reason, and a politically correct reason, it often is neither a *sufficient* nor *efficient* reason for quitting. For example, how long have you known that smoking is not good for your health.

Q. Right, right, okay. For a long time. A long, long time.

A. So you've had health reasons for quitting for a long, long time. Yet still you're smoking, so these reasons are obviously not very efficient, or sufficient.

Q. Well, they should be, though. I mean, geez, if something's going to kill you, it just makes sense not to do it.

A. But still you're doing it.

Q. Yes, okay, I see your point.

A. Let me point out that everybody —whether they are smokers or doctors --- assumes that health reasons *should* be sufficient reason to quit smoking. It's just logical that when someone finds out that what they are doing has such potentially harmful effects, they would quit doing it. But rather than looking at what *should* be or might be, what to us seems logical, let's look simply at *what is*. Let's look at the reality.

Q. The reality is that I'm a slug. I'm weak. I should have quit a long time ago.

A. No, you are not a slug. You are not weak. You are a total miracle. The way your brain synapses fire, your heart pumps, your digestion functions---you have memories and hopes for the future and warm human relationships---all of these are part of the miracle.

Q. So why do I feel like a slug?

A. Because our culture has led you to believe that reality --- your reality--- is what "should be" rather than what is.

Q. What do you mean?

A. The reality is that you have a ton of good health reasons for quitting, but you're still smoking, yes?

Q. Yes, obviously.

A. So the reality is that this ton of good health reasons for quitting has not "worked" yet to help you quit, make you quit, let you quit.

Q. Right.

A. I'm suggesting the fault --- the weakness --- is not in you. It's in the *reasons* you've been given. Again, they are deeply logical reasons, very politically correct reasons, based on a ton of research. It's not that you are unfamiliar with all the good health reasons for quitting. You may not have all the intricate details or the latest iterations, but nevertheless you have a whole warehouse full of health reasons for quitting. Waiting for more health reasons might work --- go to the doctor and get pictures of what your lungs look like, or how your heart sounds, and hear him say, "oh-oh."

Q. I don't want to wait that long.

A. Exactly. That's why I point out that health reasons, although logical and politically correct, are neither sufficient nor efficient.

Q. Okay. I see where you're going.

A. Not going anywhere. We're there!

Q. (Laughs.)

A. The easy way to *stop doing* smokes is based on *what is*, on the reality of our daily experience, rather than what *should* be.

Q. Yes. I like that. Though I admit my daily experience gives me lots of reasons --- health reasons --- for quitting.

A. Again, it's not that the health reasons aren't there, aren't real and sometimes scary. It's just that these reasons are not the most efficient, or effective way to quit smoking. There's got to be an easier way.

Q. I like that. Yes, thank you.

A. You're welcome. Should we get back on the bus, continue the adventure?

Q. Yea. Just as soon as I stop coughing.

A. (Laughs.)

Back of the Bus: Chapter 11: A Change of Lifestyle

Q. I like the idea that quitting smoking is simply a change of lifestyle. That makes the whole process seem a little less daunting. But I've engaged this old smoking lifestyle for a long, long time. Changing lifestyles to non-smoking isn't going to be all that easy.

A. The primary lifestyle that most of us have been engaging for most of our lives is the lifestyle that relies on *doing, doing, doing* in an attempt to gain more well-being. And you're right, it's not that easy to let go of a long-ingrained habit. Unless of course, we see how little well-being our *doing, doing, doing* has actually accomplished.

Q. I don't agree. If I hadn't been *doing, doing, doing* for a lot of years I probably wouldn't have my home, or my family or my job. These are a big part of my current well-being. If I hadn't been *doing, doing, doing*, I'd probably be under a bridge somewhere. Come to think of it, the *doing* lifestyle is very important to me. I don't know if I could, or would want to give it up.

A. I'm not asking you to give up *doing*. In fact, it's impossible to give up *doing*. At a very basic level you will continue to *do* your heartbeat, your breathing, your digestion, even your thinking until the moment you drop the body. This is not about giving up *doing*.

Q. So what are you asking?

A. First, I'm asking you to simply look and see whether or not your well-being actually does depend on all this *doing, doing, doing*. For example, are you totally satisfied with your home, your family, your job? You say your well-being depends on these.

Q. Yes I like these things. I love them, especially my family. All these things are mostly good. There's room for improvement, of course, especially in the job, and the money area, but in general, yea, I'm cool with my family, my home, my job. I'm satisfied with them. They're a big part of my well-being.

A. So you wake up in the morning grinning, at peace. You move through the day unhurried, enjoying yourself and the people around you. You're content, at ease, untroubled, most of the day, every day?

Q. (Laughs) Well, I wouldn't go that far.

A. Again, I'm not arguing. A home, a family, a job are all wonderful expressions of well-being. Yet most of us have not learned to deeply enjoy our well-being , or even recognize the well-being that is already present until somebody asks us about it, or reminds us. And then we will argue for it, just as you have, because it does seem very important. And yet, throughout most of our days, for most people, we have forgotten, or ignored, or diminished this very-important well-being simply because we are focusing on *doing, doing, doing,* all day long. We have been trained into this *doing, doing* lifestyle. Most of us wake in the morning with a to-do list, pressing ideas of what we need *to do* today, with the background notion that if/when we get all of these things done, our well-being will be improved, or protected.

Q. Yes, yes. I recognize that in my own life.

A. You said that your family, your home, your job were all cool, although there's room for improvement.

Q. Yea. That's true.

A. Good. I believe you. So let's look at your life as a whole --- including family, home, job, health. Just as a thought experiment, let's throw them all into one basket: here's one hundred percent of your whole life. Now, just for fun, let's try to estimate: what percent of your whole life needs improvement?

Q. What needs improvement?

A. What percentage needs improvement? We don't need to go into details. We're looking at the whole pie of your life. What percentage would you guess needs improvement?

Q. Well, everything needs improvement I guess.

A. (Laughs.) There, see, that's the basic approach to life as we've been taught it. *Could have had a much improved sunrise this morning. We could use better weather. My spouse could be richer, more beautiful, kids could be more attentive, smarter, the boss needs to pay me better*, and on and on.

Q. Yea, yea, I see where you're going.

A. For most of us, that's our habitual *lifestyle*. We're constantly trying to improve everything. Maybe not the sunrise. But often the weather. Our spouse, our kids, our home, our work. We're hoping that at some point we'll get everything just perfect. But we seldom get there. We have moments here and there, maybe on vacation, or when we complete a home project, or the kids bring home a great report card. But in general, to paraphrase Thoreau, most of us live lives of quiet anticipation that at some point down the road our well-being will be complete.

Q. Yes, you're right.

A. Curiously, as we've already talked, many people smoke because they want out of this rat race, they need a moment of well-being *right now*.

Q The *ahh* moment.
A. Exactly.

Q. I see, yes. And back to your question, when you ask me about it, and I actually stop to think about my life as a whole, I would have to say that 98% of my life is great, perfect, better than I could have imagined it back when I was young.

A. Yes. Ninety-eight percent of your life is great. What percent of the time do you remember it's great?

Q. (laughs.) Right. About two percent of the time.

A. The practice I am encouraging here --- the lifestyle I am encouraging you to experiment with --- is to take moments throughout the day to take the emphasis off of doing and *just be.* Take a moment to enjoy who you are right now, not fight the life you are living. Or more fundamentally, don't ignore the life that you are living right now, here in this moment.

Q. And this will lead to my giving up smoking?

A. This will lead to enjoying your life more. And enjoying more of your life. As we give ourselves permission to enjoy our lives more, that which we don't enjoy easily drops away. Again, it's a gentle change of lifestyle. Taking the emphasis off of *doing, doing, doing*, and putting it on *just being*.

Q. Though I can keep doing?
A. Of course.

Q. I like it.
A. That's the practice. Just relax, and like your life.

Q. (laughs.)

Back of the Bus: Chapter 12: Picking up Hitchhikers!

Q. I like where you're going with this. I like your metaphor.

A. Thanks. It's fun, isn't it? We're on a roll here. Let's just keep going.

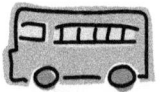

Back of the Bus: Chapter 13: Mr. T. Lives on Attention?

Q. Mr. T. lives on attention?

A. Exactly. The smoking habit is a habit of attention. Actually, all habits, all addictions, are addictions of attention. But we can just work with smoking, since this is the topic of our essay.

Q. I think I see where you're going with this. We're going to have to learn how to take our attention off of the smokes, aren't we?

A. Bingo.

Q. I'm not sure I'm going to be able to do that.

A. Actually, you do it all the time. It's very natural to *not* pick up Mr. T., the hitchhiker. But we're getting ahead of ourselves. Just watch. You don't have to *do* anything with what you're learning here, what you're seeing here. Just hang out. It's going to happen.

Q. That's good news.

A. Isn't it? (laughs.)

Back of the Bus: Chapter 14:
Waiting to Discover Mr. T.'s Other Face

Q, Okay, okay. I'm not taking time here at the back of the bus. I want to find out Mr. T.'s other face.

A. (Grins) Good. That's what I was hoping for. You're excused. Onward...

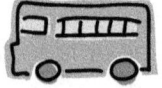

Back of the Bus: Chapter 15: Mr. T.'s Secret Face

Q. So you're telling me that my trying to quit is also the hitchhiker?

A. Yep.

Q. Geez. This is getting really complicated.

A. That's what the hitchhiker would have you believe --- that it's too complicated. But just a few chapters back you were complaining this approach was too simple, too easy.

Q. Okay. You're right. So what do I do?

A. That's the good news. You don't have to *do* anything. Nothing. Just seeing these things starts the process working on its own.

Q. Okay. Remind me again what I'm seeing.

A. That the smoking addiction is an addiction of attention. And that where attention goes, identity flows.

Q. That's clever. Where attention goes, identity flows.

A. Isn't it?

Q. So remind me again how that works.

A. Just re-read these past couple of chapters. The key here — and it really is a key to the whole process -- is that the focus of your *attention* is what creates your various identities. Seeing how this works in your own daily life will help you immensely when it comes to walking away from the hitchhiker.

Q. So give me some more examples.

A. Okay. What's your work—your profession?

Q. I'm an elementary school teacher.

A. Okay, so when you're in front of your class, you have your teacher identity on, yes?

Q. Yes, I guess you could put it that way.

A. But when you're talking with your principal, you have your co-worker, or employee identity on, yes?

Q. Yes. It's just a different aspect of my teacher identity, but I see what you mean, I think.

A. When you're talking one to one with your principal it has a different feel, a different texture, a different rhythm and tenor than when you are talking one to one with one of your students, yes?

Q. Yes. Actually, my principal thinks I'm one of her students.

A. (Laughs.) Okay, there. There's a certain irritation and tension that rises up in that relationship, that identity that isn't there when you're working with your students, right?

Q. It's a different type of tension --- and sometimes irritation—when I'm working with my students. Right. I see where you're going.

A. This may not be the best example because when you're with your principal or with your students you may be putting your attention on a particular teaching subject. Or you may see your teacher identity as part of all that. Let me ask, are you part of the teacher's union?

Q. Yes. In fact I'm one of the union representatives for our local district.

A. Okay. So let's jump to a union meeting. Do you have a different identity when you're there, talking with other representatives, and officials, than when you're in front of the classroom.

Q. Definitely. Yes. Okay. I see what you mean.

A. It's actually much simpler than we're making it here. When I share this idea with clients in my office I have them first put their attention on a philodendron that's growing there. Everybody has a slightly different story, feeling, reaction to such a common plant. For some people, it's a warm homey feeling. For others, it's bland and sad. Then I have people switch their attention to my desk lamp, which looks like a bookie's lamp. Again, people have different reactions. For some it's nice. Others wouldn't have such a lamp in the same room with them. Again, what's important to see here is the inner mechanism: *where attention goes, identity flows*.

Q. Okay. So back to the hitchhiker.

A. Let's go back even a step further... back to the smokes. Whenever you put your attention on the smokes, you bring up the hitchhiker identity. And just as you recognized with your teacher identity, the hitchhiker identity can take on many forms. The identity you have when talking with your principal and the identity you have when talking with your students are aspects of your teacher identity.

Q. Right. Okay.

A. In the same way, the hitchhiker appears as the "me" who wants to smoke and at another point the "me" who wants to quit. Both of these identities are the hitchhiker. With your school-teacher identity you can't decide, "okay, I'm just going to pay attention to my students and not pay attention to my principal," or "I'm just going to pay attention to my principal and not pay attention to my students."

Q. What a beautiful choice!

A. (Laughs) Right, but it doesn't work, does it? If you're going to give up your schoolteacher identity, you give up both. In the same way, to let go of the hitchhiker identity you let go of both the "I want to smoke" and "I want to quit" aspects of the hitchhiker.

Q. Hmm… that would take the struggle out of it, wouldn't it.

A. Bingo.

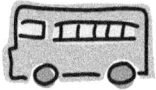

Back of the Bus: Chapter 16:
Step One of the Two Step Process

Q. Okay. It's starting to sink in. *Just be*. Don't do anything. Let happen what happens.

A. You got it.

Q. You say it's easy. But it doesn't seem that easy.

A. It actually is quite easy, and very natural to let things be the way they are, within and without. Although it's easy and natural, it's not very common. That's why it seems hard. Because we haven't been trained --- or we haven't been allowed --- to let things simply be the way they are.

Q. Right. We're constantly trying to make things better, or different, or easier.

A. You have to be brave to just let happen what's already happening, within and without. Brave, because it goes against our training, our cultural conditioning. But we fell into smoking because of our cultural conditioning. As we mature, we realize we want to be free of this old conditioning.

Q. And we do that by letting things be the way they are? That's very paradoxical.

A. Isn't it? But to let things be the way they are is actually very easy. We don't have to *do* anything. But since doing it the easy way, not doing anything is contrary to our cultural conditioning, we have to be brave. In other words, we have to be brave to let quitting be easy.

Q. (laughs.) I like it. I'd like to be brave in that way.

A. Again, although it's not very common to let things be just the way they are, is actually very natural. Kids do it all the time.

Q. So I get to be a kid again!

A. Deep down, you always were.

Q. (Is quiet.) Yes, thank you.

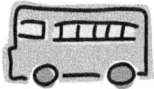

Back of the Bus: Chapter 17:
A Pause, then Change the Channel

Q. Okay, I got it. Step one is I just accept who I am, and step two is to then change the channel, move my attention.

A. That's it.

Q. What if my channel changer is busted?

A. (Laughs.)

Q. Really. I'm serious. When I try to quit smoking, I generally can't think about anything else. All I think about is smoking, smoking, smoking.

A. Yes. I'm familiar with that story. That's why I point out that the smoking addiction is at root an addiction of attention.

Q. So what do I do if I can't change the channel, can't think about anything except smoking?

A. Step one. Accept that here you are, thinking about smoking. With practice, you can take it to the next level, and *enjoy* the fact that here you are, thinking about smoking.

Q. But if I keep thinking about it, I know I'm going to do it.

A. Okay, let's allow ourselves to just look at this whole process a little more closely. The process I'm suggesting here is indeed very easy, and very natural, but in fact, contrary to our immediate assumptions, it's not very common to engage this process.

Q. What do you mean?

A. Step one, deep acceptance of who we are in the moment --- deep acceptance of what we're feeling, thinking, sensing in the moment, without fighting it, without fighting ourselves --- is *not* what we have learned, is not what most people allow themselves. More to the point, let me suggest that when you have tried to quit smoking in the past and have found that all you can think about, as you put it, is *smoking, smoking, smoking*, you were not at ease with what was arising in you in the moment.

Q. You can say that again.

A. You were not at ease with what was arising in you in the moment.

Q. (laughs.) Okay, okay. Very funny.

A. Most smokers tell themselves they *shouldn't* think about smoking. They tell themselves they *can't* think about smoking, for the exact reason you say. They worry that if they think about it too much, they'll smoke.

Q. Isn't that the case? That seems to be my experience.

A. Yes, obviously. What we put our attention on, grows. That's the magic of attention.

Q. Yes. I can see that.

A. So let's just observe what's happening. What most smokers do when trying to quit is they try to *not* think about it. So then when thoughts come up about smoking, they get irritated, try to get away from such thoughts.

Q. Isn't that exactly what you're suggesting in step two --- to change the channel?

A. Yes, you're right. That's step two. In a moment we'll talk about the difference between thinking and attention. But for now let's stick with just step one, because if we don't do step one, step two does get very, very difficult, just as you have observed.

Q. So, step one. Just accept?

A. Yes. Deep acceptance. Which means not fighting ourselves, not fighting what comes up in the moment. Basically, not trying to change ourselves --- our thoughts, feelings, sensations --- just be with them, for a moment.

Q. Okay. I think I see where you're going with this.

A. Good. Step one is based on the old principle, *what you resist, persists*. Most smokers when they try to quit try to get away from their thoughts about smoking, their feelings, their sensations. They assume that's what they are supposed to do. But that's a little bit like putting your thumb over a dripping faucet, trying to stop the drip.

Q. It's not going to happen.

A. Exactly. The same thing happens when we try *not* to think about smoking. It's like the Zen master who tells his student, "Go sit in the corner and *don't* think of a white horse." That's all the student will think about.

Q. Yea, I can see that.

A. If the student ignores the Zen Master's instructions, gives himself permission to think of the white horse, allows images of the white horse to come and go, no big deal, then fairly soon he will be thinking about what's for dinner, or the pretty Zen nun across the hall.

Q. Yes. I see.

A. Curiously, and I've worked with many smokers who confirm this observation, we often "give in" and have a smoke because it's the only way we know to finally *stop thinking* about the stupid things! When we actually have a smoke, we don't have to think about them!

Q. (Laughs.) Yes, you're right.

A. So step one is to deeply accept whatever is rising up. We don't exaggerate it or try to ignore it or change it. We simply *be with it*. Like the white horse. We let the images, the thoughts come and go.

Q. And then what about changing the channel?

A. It happens naturally. Life continues to move. Step two is we allow it to move, and then allow ourselves to get curious about what is around us, about whatever our attention happens to land upon.

Q. Like the rusty Oldsmobile.

A. Exactly. Or the light patterns on the desk. Or the sounds of the trash truck stopping and starting as it makes its way down the street.

Q. So tell me the difference between thinking and attention.

A. Yes. We can put our attention on our thoughts, and we can think about attention. To simplify, we can observe that thoughts come and go but attention remains.

Q. Okay.

A. For example, if I asked you to silently count to ten to yourself, you would hear the numbers inside your head, yes? You can try it right now and see.

Q. Yes.

A. Are you aware of the sounds of your inner voice counting?

Q. Yes.

A. So I would suggest that you are not in essence the numbers there in your head. You are that which is aware of the numbers.

Q. Okay.

A. When we are counting silently to ourselves it is generally easy to see that we are not these numbers. Or that we are more than these numbers. We are not *confined* to the numbers rising up and then disappearing in our awareness.

Q. Again, yes.

A. But most people most of the time *do* identify with the thoughts that are rising up in their awareness. And that's why most people most of the time are quite uneasy with themselves and with the world. They have identified with something fleeting, insubstantial.

Q. So relative to smoking, are you suggesting that I don't have to identify with the thoughts that are rising up about smoking?

A. Bingo, again.

Q. Wow. (pauses, obviously contemplating.) That makes it hard to even think about the whole thing!

A. (Laughs.) Exactly.

Q. So let's get back to step two. How does this tie in?

A. If you aren't so identified with your thinking, it's obviously much easier to let the thoughts come and go. Deep acceptance of what is arising in the moment --- which is step one --- is another way of saying "hands off." We're not trying to change ourselves, rearrange ourselves, make ourselves larger or smaller. We have a "hands off" attitude, or approach. We're being very friendly to ourselves when we do this. And come to find out, contrary to our training and expectations, life flows along quite naturally, quite harmoniously when we allow ourselves this "hands-off" approach to our momentary experience.

Q. I can see how that would be. And you're right, it is contrary to our training and expectations. We assume that if we aren't always grubbing around with everything, we'll be in a mess. But when we grub around, we're actually creating the mess.

A. Yes. I like your description. "Grubbing around" is another way of describing the "hands on" approach, constantly trying to change, rearrange, exaggerate or diminish our momentary experience.

Q. Hands off is step one, though. Step two?

A. Obviously, when we are taking a hands off approach --- hands off the hitchhiker --- it is then quite easy to move our attention to any of ten thousand other things.

Q. Okay. Now it is your turn. Bingo. I get it. Yes. Thank you.

A. And thank you. I think we've played a good game here. Time to move our attention elsewhere.

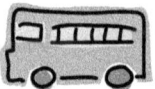

Back of the Bus: Chapter 18: The No-Big-Deal Strategy

Q. The no-big-deal strategy?
A. Yep. The no-big-deal strategy.

Q. Okay. Let's not make it a big deal. So it goes.
A. So it goes.

Q. See you after the next chapter.
A. You're catching on.

Q. No big deal.

Back of the Bus Chapter 19: What to Do With Your Smokes

Q. So you're saying don't throw my smokes away? Don't give them away? Don't smoke them up?

A. It's a matter of attention. How many do you have left?

Q. (Laughs) Okay. Actually, I just bought a new pack.

A. So now there's something at ease in your brain, yes? Something that says, I'm not quitting yet. I don't have to quit yet. I can't quit yet. I've got this pack. Maybe after this pack, or the next pack.

Q. Yes, you're right. Buying a pack buys me some time.

A. That's the hitchhiker talking. That's Mr. T. He's very quick to agree that you'll be ready to quit later, maybe even after this particular pack. You don't have to fight him, or argue with him. You don't even have to say okay, I'll quit right now. All you have to do is be aware of how he operates.

Q. As you point it out, I see that he's built up quit a story, quite a series of defenses around having smokes or not having smokes.

A. Good insight.

Q. So what do I do?

A. Again, just observe. Just be. Recognize that *not doing smokes* really doesn't depend on whether you physically have smokes or not. You can quickly observe that this planet offers you literally uncountable opportunities to get another smoke, if and when you are so inclined. Whether you do smokes or don't do smokes does not depend on whether smokes are available, near or far. They will always be available, even in jail, or at the top of the mountain.

Q. Yea, you're right. But I don't know if I can quit if I still have them around.

A. There's no hard and fast rule here. Follow your joy. You might be really glad to not physically have them in your house, or your car. Again, though, this is not at root a physical addiction. It's an addiction of attention. If you find that when you have smokes available you can't get your attention off them, it might be easier for you to not have them around. On the other hand, if you find when you don't have them you are constantly thinking about going to get a pack, you might find it easier to have them around.

Q. What if I constantly think about them whether I have them or not?

A. (Laughs) That's where all the other strategies in this book come in. Relax. Just be. Accept that you think about them all the time. The point here is that whether you have smokes or don't have smokes does not at root determine whether you *do* smokes. Whether you physically have smokes or don't have smokes is no big deal.

Q. Okay. There. That puts it into perspective. It's no big deal, one way or the other. Thank you.

A. You're welcome. No big deal.

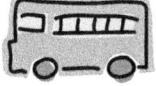

Back of the Bus: Chapter 20: Hook Me Up, Doc

Q. I tried the patches and found they gave me a rash. So I can't use them.

A. I've heard that a lot. The good news is that you don't really need them in order to *stop doing* the smokes. Nevertheless, if you're still wanting to experiment with the patch, you may want to try different brands. Most often the rash is a reaction to the adhesive, not the nicotine. Different brands use different adhesives.

Q. When using these products, aren't we just exchanging one addiction for another? We're still addicted to nicotine.

A. Actually, if I may refresh your memory, our primary addiction is not to the nicotine, but to the pause that refreshes, the *ahh*, the brief moment in smoking where we give ourselves a break from *doing, doing, doing*.

Q, Yea, yea.

A. (Laughs.) I appreciate your frustration but this is not a minor point. If it was primarily an addiction to nicotine --- which most smokers assume --- then the patches, gum or lozenges would work to help us stop doing smokes seventy, eighty, ninety percent of the time.

Unfortunately, the numbers for success are about reverse this.

Q. What, only a ten to thirty percent rate?

A. Alas, yes. Those are the figures. On the lower end by independent researchers, the higher end for the studies funded by pharmaceutical companies.

Q. Okay, granted. Thanks for reminding me. But still, aren't we running the risk of becoming addicted to these things?

A. Yes, it happens, especially with the gum or lozenges. It's very rare that someone becomes addicted to the patches.

Q. What's the diff?

A. With the patches, we put them on once a day and forget about it. With the gum or lozenges, people often turn to them in response to a craving, which is the same thing they were doing with the smokes. *Ahh*, another lozenge.

Q. Okay. That makes sense. So again, aren't we running the risk of exchanging one addiction for another?

A. Yes, we are, again, especially with the gum and lozenges. Nevertheless, the powers that be still encourage these products because the real harm from smoking does not come from the nicotine, but rather from the four thousand other chemicals that are released when you combust tobacco.

Q. So it's better to be addicted to the gum or lozenges than to the smokes.

A. Yes, much, much better. So don't let this be a big concern. On the other hand, none of us want to be addicted to anything. My experience is that most folks using the gum or lozenges get to a point where they are simply tired of it. They don't want the hassle. And walk away from it very naturally.

Q. That's good news.

A. Practice just being and deeply accepting yourself in the moment. Your freedom will grow, as will your peace and joy. Just be, you'll see.

Q. Thank you.

A. *Da nada.*

Back of the Bus: Chapter 21: Better Living through Chemistry

Q. So, spit it out: are you for or against using Zyban?
A. Yes.

Q. Right. Let me guess. For it when somebody wants to try it. Against it if they don't.
A. Exactly.

Q. Okay. Let me put it another way. If you were still trying to quit smoking, would you try it?
A. Probably. It seems like I tried everything to quit before I finally did. I confess, I'm an old geezer. I stopped doing my smokes before the FDA approved Zyban as a stop smoking aid. Knowing my mindset at the time, I probably would have tried Zyban, then probably would have found I enjoyed its relaxing psychological effects, then became addicted to it while I continued to smoke a pack a day.

Q. (Laughs.) Yea. I can dig it.
A. But let me be clear. Zyban wasn't available, so I didn't personally use Zyban, nor did I

become addicted to it. Back then, though, I was like most of my generation. We were looking for something we could *do* to achieve well-being, and we were fortunate enough to be in the era where we at least recognized that the "doing" to achieve well-being was related to our inner mental processes rather than outer accumulations.

Q. Turn on, tune in, drop out.

A. You're quoting Saint Timothy. That era didn't last very long, even for the people who were in it. The worldwide belief system that suggests we can *do* something ---*do, do, do*--- to achieve well-being was too strong, had too much momentum. We, too, were infected. So most of us stopped looking within and starting marching again in lock-step --- or at least dance-step --- with the worldwide belief that we could find something to *do* that would create well-being.

Fortunately, here in the new millennium, there's a new era dawning. Many of us--- regardless of age or background--- are starting to recognize that well-being is already present, already closer than our very breath, if we just take a moment to acknowledge it.

Q. So knowing what you know now, in your present mindset, you probably wouldn't use Zyban?

A. No. probably not. I'm too jealous, and protective of my simple ordinary mind, or more specifically, my ordinary being, in which the mind rises and falls. I'm finally starting to recognize what a miracle it is, just to be awake, alive, present, aware, going to the grocery store.

Q. (Laughs.) Yes, thank you.

A. Again, let me be clear. For some folks, that simple, ordinary every-day wakefulness, everyday awareness, might indeed include a curiosity and openness to trying Zyban. That's what arises in them. So be it. Let them experiment. Let them explore. Being itself allows all possibilities. No blame there. My experience is that at some point we tire of being's possibilities --- which are infinite --- and become curious, fascinated, with being itself. That's when the prodigal son turns around and heads home.

Q. Umm… yes. I get it. Home, which is being itself.

A. Yes. Being itself. Being itself is the most powerful drug in the universe. If you let it, being itself will cure what ails you.

Q. I believe it. Thank you.

A. You're welcome. This outer voice is your own inner being, calling you home.

Q. Stop! Stop! I cant take it any more.

A. (Laughs.) Me neither. Sometimes I wax too poetic. Let's go look at Chantix, another drug.

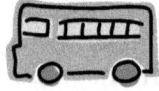

Back of the Bus: Chapter 22: Chantix: Like Smoking a Carrot

Q. So let me ask the same question I asked about Zyban. Would you recommend Chantix? Or would you yourself take it?

A. No, to both questions. Though again, the qualifier --- if you're curious, give it a shot. It probably won't kill you, though it might.

Q. (laughs.) Yikes! It might?

A. Heart problems and suicidal ideations are part of the documented risks of Chantix. But welcome to earth. Walking out in front of a bus could also kill us. Drinking too much coffee --- who knows. We've discovered and deeply documented that what we do here on planet earth seems to kill us.

Q. Okay, yes. Granted. But for a stop smoking aid, would you recommend it?

A. Again, no. But I'm a realist. I know that for some people my suggestion to simply rest in their ordinary being, accept themselves just as they are, accept whatever arises, is too simple, too seemingly airy-fairy, though in fact this approach is as nuts and bolts real as it gets. Nevertheless, as mentioned, I've had several friends, long-term clients who for one reason or another weren't able to stop doing their smokes and then when they took Chantix they finally were able to stop doing their smokes. Chantix gave them the excuse, or the mindset or the opportunity to do what they'd been wanting to do for a long time... which is to *not do anything* about their smokes. So in those cases I'd give Chantix the credit.

Q. Are these people still smoke-free?

A. Good question. I've lost contact with the two or three that claimed success using Chantix. I'll give them the benefit of the doubt, and assume they have remained abstinent. I've had many other clients who tried Chantix and did not succeed, or had to stop taking it because they couldn't stand the side-effects.

As you might suspect, I think there's an easier way. And the deep invasiveness and uncertainty of the outcome for Chantix makes me hesitate to recommend it. Again, though, *being* itself is wide open. *Being* cradles all possibilities. Chantix is one of those possibilities. If folks are curious, want to give it a try, so be it.

For folks who do want to try Chantix, I would encourage them to bring their family and friends in on the deal. Ask family or friends to monitor what's going on and to let them know when or if they start acting violent or depressed. Chantix does, after all, have the reputation for inciting more violent acts than any other prescription drug. Meth undoubtedly elicits more violence, but it's hard to get a prescription for meth.

Q. Your position is pretty clear. Maybe we should just leave it at that.

A. Thanks. Let's move on to something easier.

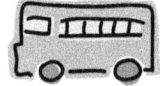

Back of the Bus: Chapter 23: Improvise!

Q. Improvise. Just make it up, huh? Just fake it?
A. That's it.

Q. Seems almost too easy.
A. Almost.

Q. That takes the pressure off. I like it.
A. I thought you might.

Q. Okay. If I can just fake it, make it up, I don't need to ask any questions.
A. Perfect.

Q. Except for maybe just one.
A. Shoot.

Q. If I just need to fake it, make it up as I go along, why do I need this book?
A. (Laughs). Bingo. You don't. You never did. That's what this book helps you to see!

Back of the Bus: Chapter 24: Set a Quit Date or Not?

Q. So, you're suggesting *not* to set a quit date?

A. That's not what I said. But let's look. Have you set one before?

Q. Yes.

A. And you're still smoking?

Q. Yes.

A. Hmm….

Q. But if I don't set a quit date won't I just continue to smoke forever, then?

A. Is that what you want to do?

Q. No. I want to quit.

A. Okay. Just be with that for a moment, if I can refresh your memory as to our approach here. You say you just want to quit—you just want to *stop doing* smokes.

Q. Yes.

A. So just be with that. Just for a moment, don't try to figure out *how* or *where* or *when*. Rather, just be with what rises up in you, which is that you want to quit. You don't need to exaggerate it. You don't need to make it larger than it is. Or smaller, either one. Just *be* with it --- be with the honest feeling that you don't want to do smokes. Feel it as it rises up in you. You don't have to *do* anything about it. Just be with it.

Q. Okay. But how do I do it? How do I actually quit?

A. *This* is how you do it. Stop *doing* for a moment and *just be* with your own true, deep, honest feelings, with your own self. In this moment your feelings are that you really don't want to do smokes any more. So for a moment, don't worry about *how* you're going to stop doing smokes. Rather, for a moment just feel how it is to be yourself --- your plain, ordinary, every-day self --- here in this moment. Just be with the experience, the feeling that you want to stop doing smokes.

Q. Yes, okay. But I've wanted to quit for longer than I care to admit. Years and years. Just being with wanting to quit is what I've been doing.

A. Careful, now. Let's work with your direct experience, not your intellectual ideas of your experience. Have you ever truly just sat, so to speak, with the feeling of not wanting to smoke, without at the same time immediately trying to figure out how to *do* it? Or when to *do* it?

Q. Okay. I see what you mean. No, probably not. As soon as I feel I want to quit, I either try to figure out how to do it, or, more often, just drop it because I can't figure it out. It's too big of a problem.

A. Right. That's why this very simple, very easy suggestion of *just being* with your ordinary self, without trying to change it, without trying to fix it, is actually a very new approach for most smokers. The old approach is, *what can I do, what can I do, what can I do to fix me?* The good news is, you don't need fixing!

Q. Yes, thank you. That feels right. I can see that. And as you say it, as I start to do it -- start to *just be* with whatever arises -- it feels pretty good. So you're saying if I *just be* with this feeling of wanting to quit...

A. You're just being with yourself. You're coming home. Coming home to yourself.

Q. Again, okay. I see that. And you're suggesting that if I do that enough I'll quit smoking?

A. What do you have to *do* to just be with yourself? Just be with your feelings?

Q. (Laughs.) Nothing.

A. And what have I been saying, again, and again and again, as to the easiest approach to *not doing* smokes? What do we have to *do* to not do smokes?

Q. Nothing!

A. Again. Bingo.

Q. Okay. But the problem is that maybe for a moment I will just be with the feeling I want to quit. But then the feeling that I want to have a smoke comes up. And it's a lot stronger than the feeling of wanting to quit.

A. Okay. So just be with that feeling when it arises. There's no work here. Just be with who you are in the moment.

Q. Yea, but then I'll smoke.

A. Maybe, maybe not.

Q. The last twenty years or more would suggest that I will.

A. Have you been doing this practice, which is really no practice for the last twenty years? Have you consistently accepted all of your feelings, without trying to escape? Have you come to terms with your ordinary self, so that you enjoy your own company, are not constantly trying to fix yourself?

Q. Okay. No. That has not been my practice.

A. You noticed that the urge to not do smokes rises up. And then it also goes away, yes?

Q. Yes. That's the problem.

A. No. It's not a problem. Your ordinary experience is reality. It's not a problem. Our invitation here is to cease making our ordinary experience into a problem.

Q. Okay, yes. Thank you.

A. So we've noticed that the urge to not do smokes rises up and then falls away. And I'm suggesting we don't have to *do* anything about that. In the same way, the urge to do smokes rises up, and then it too falls away. We don't have to *do* anything about that, either.

Q. Ahh, okay. I see.

A. Let's go back to setting a quit date as an example. Setting a quit date is based on the notion that what rises up in our ordinary being on that date will be easier to manage than what rises up in our ordinary being right now. And right now, the urge, the notion, the command to set a quit date rises up. And then the reaction against setting a quit date rises up.

Q. Yes. I see that very clearly in me.

A. For some folks, the idea of setting a quit date is very welcome, natural, easy. So they follow that path. For others, it's not. We're learning here not to fight ourselves. It's a little bit like learning to not fight it when Uncle Louie wants to give us a thousand dollars, no strings attached. Okay. It's a delicious learning process. Except learning to not fight ourselves is even more valuable than a thousand dollars. It's a million dollar gift.

Q. I can see that. But like you say, it's not what we were taught.

A. No. Generally not. What we were taught led us to *do* smoking. It's time to let go of the old ways of relating to ourselves, which is to always try to fix ourselves, and instead to begin to love ourselves, be at peace with ourselves, listen to ourselves just as we are, and honor that. **If we aren't free to simply be ourselves, here in the moment, just as we are, we won't ever be free**.

Q. Wow. Yes. I can see that.

A. But we *are* free to be ourselves, here in the moment. Nobody anywhere can take this freedom away. It's our inherent freedom. It's like the color of our eyes. As we allow ourselves to be just who we are, deeply accept who we are in the moment, our chains fall away.

Q. Like the chains of smoking.
A. Bingo.

Q. You're a damned poet, you know that?
A. (laughs.) And my feet show it. They're Longfellows!

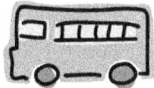

Back of the Bus: Chapter 25: Nourish the Inner Slacker

Q. So that's it, huh? It boils down to just being a slacker?
A. That's it. Bingo.

Q. Seems almost too easy.
A. Almost.

Q. But it makes sense. I like it.
A. Good. I was hoping you would.

Q. Thank you for taking the time to do this with us. And for these question and answer sessions here at the back of the bus. They've really helped.
A. Glad to hear it. And you're welcome. I tell people I really enjoy my work because I basically get to remind people what they already know. It makes my job easy.

Q. (Laughs) Yea, you're right. We really do already know all this stuff, don't we?
A. Yes.

Q. It's nice to be reminded.
A. It's fun to remind.

Q. I'm going to go off now and be a slacker.
A. Me, too.

Q. Slackers unite!
A. It takes too much energy.

Q. (Laughs.) Thanks.
A. You're welcome. Peace to you, friend. Who you already are is already enough.

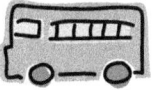

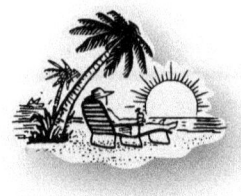 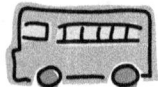

Conclusion, (Again): The Easy Exit Off Ramp

Again, sorry to say, happy to say, that's it, folks. The bus ride's over. We're back here at the Easy Exit Off Ramp. This is where we got on. This is where we get off.

As you can see, we never actually left it. The Off Ramp has always been right here in front of our nose. It was so close most of us missed it because it was that easy to overlook. Come to find out, we don't have to *do* anything to not do smokes. We don't have to go anywhere than where we are right now. We don't have to be anybody different than we are right now. When it comes to fixing ourselves, we can just be slackers. Enjoy the day. Enjoy the fresh air. Enjoy the freedom.

Easy, yes?

Glad to have had you aboard. Glad to have you exit. Feel free to contact me! I'd love to hear your stories, your questions and even your complaints. I'd especially love to hear your stories about quitting.   Contact me :

Bear Gebhardt, Head Coach,
Smoker's Freedom School
(smokersfreedomschool.com)
606 Hanna St. Fort Collins, CO. 80521
 bear@smokersfreedomschool.com

In peace.... Bear

"I see the poem or novel ending with an open door."
                              --- Michael Ondaatje

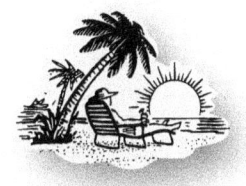

www.ingramcontent.com/pod-product-compliance
Lightning Source LLC
Chambersburg PA
CBHW070637050426
42451CB00008B/200